DISEASES AND PARASITES OF HORSES & MULES

DISEASES AND PARASITES OF HORSES & MULES

Editor
Gove Hambidge

BIOTECH

2022
Biotech Books

Original Title: Livestock Yearbook of Agriculture, 1942

ISBN10 81-7622-084-1
ISBN13 978-81-7622-084-2

Published by : **BIOTECH BOOKS**
4762-63/23, Ansari Road, Darya Ganj,
New Delhi - 110002
Phones : 011 4300 3222
Email : biotechbooks@yahoo.co.in

PRINTED IN INDIA

CONTENTS

INTRODUCTION

Equine Encephalomyelitis

This brain disease of horses has received a great deal of attention from research workers during the past few years for three reasons:

(1) The virus is capable of causing an encephalitis, or inflammation of the brain, known as sleeping sickness, in human beings; there were over 2,000 cases of encephalitis in five Western States in 1941.

(2) Since 1930 the equine disease has gradually spread east ward until it now practically blankets the entire country.

(3) During this period nearly a milllon horses and mules have been attacked by the disease.

Here are some of the facts about encephalomyelitis (which means literally inflammation of the brain and spinal cord) discussed by Giltner and Shahan:

It is now known that there are two types of virus, an eastern and a western, that produce the disease. The eastern type causes death in about 9 out of 10 cases, the western type usually in only 1 out of 4 or 5 cases.

The symptoms in a horse or mule include fever, sleepiness, stupor, grinding of the teeth, uncoordinated and wobbly movements, and difficulty in chewing and swallowing. Body functions become more or less paralyzed and ultimately the animal collapses, lying in a stupor or delirium, and dies. In some cases, however, the disease stops with the early fever stage, and it might be thought that the animal was suffering only from some other mild illness. Both types of attack confer considerable immunity.

The disease occurs in epizootics (the animal equivalent of epidemics) during the warm months is essentially confined to pastured animals, and is most common where there is water or marshy land. Every indication points to the fact that it is spread by bloodsucking insects. Experiments have proved that several species of mosquitoes and the Rocky Mountain spotted fever tick can transmit the virus, and It has been found in the field in one species of mosquito and in the assassin bug. It has also been proved that over 20 species of birds, as well as cattle, swine, sheep, goats., dogs, cats, guinea pigs, rabbits, monkeys, rats, mice, gophers, hedgehogs, and woodchucks can be infected, and since 1938 the virus has been definitely found in cases of brain disease in human beings. In fact, so far as is known, ho other virus is capable of infecting so many different species of animals.

Diagnosis of the disease is based on clinical symptoms, post mortem examination, and sometimes inoculation of laboratory animals or a neutralization test with serum. Control measures which should be carried out by a qualified veterinarian, include:

(1) Vaccination before the epizootic season with a vaccine prepared from artificially infected chick-embryo tissue treated with formaldehyde to destroy its ability to produce the disease. (An antiserum may be used, but the vaccine is usually preferable).

(2) Control of bloodsucking insects by all practicable means; in particular, protection of affected animals against these insects.

(3) Extermination of rats, mice, and other vermin and exclusion of pigeons and stray animals from the premises.

(4) Prompt and thorough disposal of animals dead of the disease, and thorough disinfection of their quarters.

Medicinal or other treatments may be used by the veterinarian to relieve certain symptoms in a sick animal. The caretaker's job is to follow instructions and do everything possible to keep the animal comfortable.

Various other diseases, some of which affect the brain, may be confused with encephalomyelitis, including moldy corn poisoning, plant poisoning, tick paralysis, anthrax, shipping fever, swamp fever, rabies, heat stroke, brain tumors and abscesses, mechanical injuries, botulism, azoturia, and an acute, highly fatal malady called toxic hepatogenous icterus which seems to follow encephalomyelitis in some areas.

Equine Infectious Anemia

As Stein points out, infectious anemia of horses, mules; and asses–also known as swamp fever, malarial fever, and by other names–has become a problem of world-wide concern. In the past 10 years out-breaks have occurred in 17 States in this country.

Caused by a virus, the disease may be either acute and rapidly fatal or, more commonly, chronic and characterized by intermittent attacks of fever (each lasting several days), loss of weight, progressive weakness, marked depression, and dropsical swellings. During and immediately after the fever there is a reduction in the number of red corpuscles in the blood, and postmortem examination frequently shows internal hemorrhages and damage to the spleen, liver, kidneys, and heart. In most areas the disease is confined to low-lying, swampy, or wooded sections, but in the Mississippi Delta it is widespread, principally in the chronic form, sapping the strength of large numbers of mules and making them incapable of work when they are most needed.

How infectious anemia spreads is not definitely known, in spite of considerable experimenting. Biting insects may play an important part; so may feed and water contaminated by the virus-laden excretions of infected animals; so may long-continued, intimate contact of infected with normal animals. It is definitely known that after recovering from an attack, animals can carry the disease in a latent form for many years, serving as unrecognized sources of infection for other animals. Diagnosis is difficult, since the symptoms can easily be confused with those of various other diseases and of parasitic infestations. The only positive means of diagnosis is to inoculate a well horse with material from the suspected case. Nor is there any medicinal treatment that will bring about a cure or any method of preventing the disease by vaccination. Control depends primarily on the identification of carriers.. Stein suggests the following steps as having practical value:

(1) Destroy any animal proved to have infectious anemia and dispose of the carcass by deep burial or cremation. (This is not practicable, of course, in regions like the Mississippi Delta, where the disease is widespread in a chronic form).

(2) Where infected animals are to be kept and worked, separate them from healthy animals and carry out all practicable steps to prevent transmission of the disease to the latter.

(3) Do not breed infected mares, since they can transmit the disease to their offspring.

(4) Plow and fence off badly contaminated pastures or other areas and exclude horses and mules from them for at least 6 months.

(5) Provide good sanitation, control intestinal parasites and flies, supply pure, fresh drinking water, and never permit animals to drink from stagnant pools.

Periodic Ophthalmia of Horses

According to some estimates, 10 percent of the horses and mules in the United States are affected with periodic ophthalmia, with the figure running as high as 30 percent in some areas. Known for 2,000 years and the subject of considerable scientific research, the disease is still a mystery from the standpoint of cause, method of spread, cure, and prevention. Primarily a disease of the eyes, it is characterized by sudden recurring attacks of inflammation, which may affect only one eye or both and may extend over a period of several years. Symptoms include swollen, tender lids, a watery discharge from the eyes, some rise in body temperature, and cloudiness of the fluid within the eye and usually of the cornea. In this disease there are usually many successive attacks, all of which are acute. Blindness is the usual termination, but it may occur very early–for example, during the first, attack. Diagnosis of the disease is not easy.

Mott and Seibold discuss the world distribution of periodic ophthalmia in some detail; a peculiarity is that it apparently seldom occurs in high attitudes. They also discuss several theories that have been advanced as to the cause of the malady. Little that is definite can be said, though the disease appears to be infectious, and possibly susceptibility to it may be inherited. Recently the Bureau of Animal Industry made a careful study of the microscopic changes in the eye that result from periodic ophthalmia, and these are described in detail by the authors.

In the absence of more definite knowledge, the best practical advice that can be given is (1) to obtain veterinary services promptly if an attack occurs, so that the animal's sight may be prolonged; (2) to keep healthy horses and mules isolated from any possible contact with animals affected by the disease; (3) not to breed animals that have the disease.

Glanders

An ancient disease of horses, mules, and asses, glanders can do an immense amount of damage, especially where these animals are concentrated in large numbers; over 58,000 had it in the French Army alone during the last war, and many of them had to be slaughtered. Occasionally other animals and human beings get the disease. Fortunately, glanders has now been practically eradicated in the United States; but as Cole points out, vigilance in excluding it from the country is all the more necessary for that reason.

The disease, which may be either acute or chronic, is caused by the germ *Bacillus mallei*. The outstanding symptom is the formation of nodules and ulcers in the nasal cavity and respiratory passages, almost always in the lungs, which are seriously affected, and sometimes in and under the skin. (The skin form of the disease is called farcy). Few animals ever recover.

A serum test, an animal inoculation test, or a mallein test-made by putting a few drops of culture into the eye–can be used for accurate diagnosis; the last is the one most commonly employed because of its simplicity and reliability. Since there is no cure for the disease and no known way of conferring immunity, positive reactors should be destroyed, all exposed animals should be promptly tested, and premises and equipment should be adequately disinfected. Many States require prompt reporting of suspected cases and pay indemnities for animals destroyed under official supervision.

Dourine

Dourine is essentially an equine syphilis caused by one of the microscopic parasites called trypanosomes and transmitted by sexual contact. As Cole points out, the first symptoms, which appear on the sex organs, may be entirely unnoticed. Secondary symptoms, appearing some time later, consist of wheals like hives, on various parts of the body. Months or even years after the disease first strikes, it may give rise to marked disturbances of the central nervous system which when end in paralysis and death. A mortality rate of 50 percent is not uncommon. There is no known cure.

Since 1912, when a serum test made it possible to diagnose cases positively, great progress has been made in eradicating the disease in this country, and it now exists only in restricted areas in three States. Serum samples, which must be prepared by an expert, are tested by the Bureau of Animal Industry. All animals with a positive test are destroyed, and the owners are indemnified.

Miscellaneous Diseases of Equines

Mott, Shahan, Giltner, and Frank deal with a considerable number of diseases of the horse, mule, and ass, for the most part not discussed elsewhere in this book.

Influenza (also called shipping fever and by other names)—Probably this is the most contagious and widely distributed disease of equines. The death rate is not especially high, but losses due to the incapacitating of work animals are serious. The disease is caused by a virus and is sometimes complicated by bacterial invasions; overwork, undue exposure, and poor hygiene are predisposing factors. Typical symptoms include fever, weakness, depression, rapid breathing, a harsh cough, watery discharges from eyes and nose, inflamed conjunctiva (pinkeye). Pneumonia, paralysis, or other serious complications may ensue. Preventive measures include quarantine of incoming animals, injections of bacterins for animals going to market (there are no specific vaccines or serums as yet, however), isolation of sick animals, disinfection of premises and equipment. Treatment consists mainly in rest and good nursing, with such medication as a veterinarian may recommend.

Distemper (Strangles)—Probably caused by a streptococcus germ, distemper presents early symptoms somewhat like those described for influenza. In most cases there is a hot, painful swelling of the submaxillary glands (under the Jaw); abscesses may form in other glands and tissues, and pneumonia and septicemia may be complications. Predisposing factors are like those for influenza. Affected animals should be, isolated and carefully nursed, and premises and equipment should be disinfected. Various treatments may be prescribed by the veterinarian, including the placing of a tube in the windpipe to prevent suffocation, Preventive measures may include the use of a bacterin and the quarantining of newly purchased animals.

Purpura hemorrhagica (*petechial fever*) is not contagious and the cause is unknown, but it seldom occurs except after severe septic infection. Hemorrhages, edema (watery swellings), a rapid pulse, and jaundice are among the usual symptoms. Serious complications are common. Veterinary treatment is directed toward alleviating symptoms.

Wounds and wound infections, which occur very commonly among horses, can cause serious trouble. The germs of tetanus, or lockjaw, are widely distributed; so are streptococci, staphlyococci, and other organisms. Whether an infection remains localized or spreads throughout the body depends on the animal's resistance at the time

and the number and character of the germs. Much of the damage from this cause is preventable by following out the management practices suggested in this article to keep animals from acquiring wounds in the first place, and by giving injuries prompt and proper care when they do occur. The article outlines first-aid treatment for wounds, describes the steps taken by the veterinarian, and in particular includes an account of the symptoms, prevention, and treatment of tetanus.

Breeding troubles frequently result from carelessness and ignorance in the handling of animals. Good diet, housing, and sanitation and proper exercise are the major preventives, but specific procedures should also be carried out in connection with breeding. These authors briefly describe the anatomy and physiology of the genital organs, and point out the need for keeping records of the heat period of mares, which varies among individuals from 12 to 30 hours. Since the egg is released near the end of the heat period, and the male sperm remains alive only 12 to 48 hours (varying among individuals), accurate timing of breeding operations is essential.

Good breeding hygiene demands a rather elaborate programme that includes veterinary examination of the mare at intervals between heat periods to determine whether there is infection or any abnormal condition of the ovaries or uterus and laboratory examination of the semen of the stallion. The actual breeding operation, which may be by normal mating or artificial insemination, demands extreme hygienic precautions to eliminate any possibility of infection. Pregnancy can be determined by manual examination or by the injection of blood serum from the mare into laboratory animals.

Abortion is due to various causes, including the effects of certain drugs (some worm medicines, for instance), poisons, certain illnesses, injuries, and infections. Streptococci are said to cause 25 percent of all abortions in mares. Contagious equine abortion, caused by a specific *Salmonella* organism, may be largely controlled by the elimination of reacting animals as breeders and the vaccination of pregnant mares. There are indications that many abortions of unknown cause are due to a specific virus.

Difficult labor, the authors point out, may result in the death of both foal and dam and calls for prompt veterinary attention. Retained placenta (afterbirth) may also have very serious consequences.

Diseases of newborn foals are due chiefly to infection, though parasitism, poor nutrition, and poor housing are also important factors. One or more of several different micro-organisms may be involved, acquired for the most part through the uterus of the dam or the umbilicus of the foal after birth. The fact that these infections are so often fatal before any treatment (even if one is available) can be effective throws special emphasis on the need for adequate breeding hygiene carried out by veterinarians rather than laymen, and for proper disinfection of the umbilical stump of the newborn foal. Drugs, serums, bacterins, and blood transfusions, however, are useful in some cases.

Lameness, of course, is particularly important in the case of equines. It should seldom occur if animals are given good care, are free from hereditary defects or seriously inferior conformation, and are properly trained and properly harnessed. Immediate attention should be given to the slightest lameness, the animal should be rested, and an accurate diagnosis should be made. The treatments used in addition to rest depend on the nature and extent of the trouble.

There are many causes and forms of lameness, of which the following are some of the more common:

(1) Sprains are a stretching, laceration, or actual rupture of tissues due to strains that may occur in a great many ways.

A sprain may result in serious injury to a joint ultimate invasion by bacteria, and such abnormalities as "bowed tendons," "bucked shins," "water knee."

(2) Arthritis is an inflammation of a joint caused by injury and sometimes complicated by bacterial infection.

(3) A luxation, or dislocation, is the displacement of a bone from its normal position–most frequently, the patella, in the stifle joint. It requires prompt treatment by special manipulation.

(4) Injury to the nerves may cause lameness, paralysis and in some cases the muscular wasting known as sweeny.

(5) Inflammation of the blood vessels or the formation of blood clots (thrombosis) caused by parasites or by injury may lead to lameness.

(6) Fractures, or broken bones, may result from severe injury or strain. In very few cases and only under ideal conditions can they be treated successfully.

(7) Stringhalt, or springhalt, which takes the form of spasmodic contractions of the muscles of the hind leg, is sometimes treated by the severing of nerves or tendons. The cause is unknown.

Bone diseases are probably the most common cause of lay-offs of draft horses and mules. They are due to faulty feeding (especially a lack of mineral balance in the diet) and to hereditary defects, with strains, injuries, and improper shoeing as contributing factors. The diseases discussed in this article are bone spavin, an enlargement of the hock bones; ringbone, an enlargement of the bones immediately below the fetlock; sidebones, a hardening of certain important cartilages on each side of the foot; splints, an abnormal growth of bone between the cannon bone and the small splint bones; navicular disease, an inflammation involving a joint within the forefoot; and the nutritional diseases, rickets and bighead, associated with calcium, phosphorus, and vitamin D metabolism. In some cases, the authors point out, specially designed shoes and appropriate trimming of the hoofs can compensate for bone deformities enough to make an animal serviceable. The whole problem of bone diseases emphasizes the need for good nutrition and a thorough understanding of conformation.

Foot ailments-After describing the structure of the foot in some detail, the authors discuss a number of foot ailments and their causes and treatment. Chief causes of foot troubles are faulty conformation and improper care of the feet, including stabling on too dry floors or in wet and filth. The following specific ailments are dealt with but cannot be more than mentioned in this brief summary:

(1) Brittle hoof is an abnormally dry, hard state of the horn, often treated by special trimming and a suitable ointment.

(2) In spongy hoof the horn is abnormally soft, and shoeing must be done with great care.

(3) In crooked foot, one side wall is higher than the other. Special shoes are sometimes used to compensate for the unevenness.

(4) A contracted foot is sometimes benefited by special shoes or by leaving the animal unshod.

(5) Sand cracks, or splits in the hoof, call for expert treatment of various kinds, depending on the location and extent of the cracks.

(6) Corns, due to changes in the tissue as a result of bruising, may be dry, moist, or suppurating. Treatment is not always satisfactory.

(7) Thrush is a diseased condition of the tissues caused by infection and nearly always produces lameness. It requires antiseptic treatment.

(8) Canker, a diseased condition that may cause the growth of a fun-goid mass instead of normal horn, usually calls for surgery and other special treatments.

(9) Grease heel, an inflammation of the skin of the pastern and fetlock, calls for antiseptic treatment and sometimes surgery.

(10) Quittor is a discharge of pus in the region of the coronary band caused by infection. Most cases require a radical surgical operation.

Skin diseases are often due directly or indirectly to faulty nutrition, unsanitary surroundings, and lack of regular grooming. Accurate diagnosis is the first step in successful treatment, but it may be difficult and require laboratory examinations. If a communicable skill disease is suspected, the animal should at once be isolated pending a diagnosis. Prescription and application of medicinal agents should be left to a veterinarian.

In addition to discussing briefly such conditions as excessive sweating, failure to sweat, so-called sweating of blood, and dandruff, the authors go into more detail regarding the following diseases:

(1) Eczema, an eruption with more or less severe itching;

(2) Acne, an inflammation of the hair follicles and sebaceous glands caused by pus-forming bacteria;

(3) Urticaria, or hives, which may be due to anyone of several causes, including a reaction to certain substances in feeds;

(4) Light sensitisation, manifested in white-skinned and white-spotted animals and apparently induced by the eating of certain plants;

(5) Ring-worm, a contagious disease caused by microscopic molds;

(6) Lymphangitis, an inflammation of the lymph vessels, which produces symptoms resembling those of glanders and is of three types–sporadic (essentially dietary in origin), ulcerative (due to bacterial infection), and mycotic (due to fungus infection).

Abnormalities of the teeth-Alveolar periostitis, an inflammation of the tissue (periosteum) that attaches the tooth to the socket (alveolus) in the jawbone, caused by food particles and infective materials that gain entrance to the alveolus, calls for prompt extraction of the affected tooth. Uneven teeth, which may lead to serious injury to the mouth and to malnutrition, may be remedied by appropriate cutting or filing.

Fistula of the withers and poll evil–These maladies are essentially the same except that they affect the withers and the poll, respectively. They involve a deep-seated, chronic inflammation of structures associated with the spine, possibly due originally to injuries caused by blows or pressure. A thread like worm has been recovered from the tissues in many cases. It is now thought that the germ responsible for brucellosis of cattle may be associated with the disease. Control measures include avoidance of injury from such causes as low feed racks and ill-adjusted collars, sometimes internal medication, careful surgery where necessary, the elimination of brucellosis in cattle and swine.

Diseases connected with management–The authors list the following troubles as due directly to mismanagement:

(1) Azoturia (black water, Monday morning disease) is characterized by a sudden stiffening and paralysis of the muscles, profuse sweating, and very dark urine. It usually appears in working animals kept on full feed during a period of rest. Treatment, if the animal is to be saved, demands immediate rest on the spot where the attack occurs and the prompt services of a veterinarian.

(2) Heaves (broken wind, asthma) is a chronic respiratory disease characterized by difficult breathing and dry cough. The condition is associated with the feeding of damaged roughage. Proper feeding will control mild cases, but little can be done once the lungs are extensively involved.

(3) Colic is a symptom of any one of about a dozen disorders of the stomach and intestines, caused most frequently by faulty feeding, overwork, exposure, and other preventable factors. Treatment is variable and should be prescribed by a veterinarian.

(4) Founder (laminitis) is a serious ailment of the feet, chiefly caused by gross overeating, with extreme pain and fever as the principal symptoms. Treatment requires the services of a veterinarian. In advanced cases little can be done except suitable shoeing.

(5) Collar and saddle sores result from failure to harden the animal gradually to work, lack of regular grooming, ill-fitting harness.

(6) Poisoning usually results from the consumption of such substances as arsenical and lead preparations, commonly used in farm operations. Symptoms and treatment are described by the authors.

Internal Parasites of Horses and Mules

Horses, mules and donkeys "provide shelter and subsistence"–as Foster puts it-for about 150 different internal parasites, which are of two kinds, the protozoa, or minute one-celled animals, and the worms, or helminths. Practically speaking, it can be said that no horse or mule is ever entirely free of internal parasites of some kind. Some of these parasites are confined to certain geographic regions; others are found everywhere. Many are highly specialized in the parts of the body they attack; some do a good deal of wandering in the body, often following certain regular routes. Thus practically every organ of the body has its parasites. The importance of these enemies is not generally recognized, partly because the damage they do is seldom in the nature of a specific or spectacular disease; rather it is a general sapping of the animal's vitality and efficiency.

In general, the protozoa are of two types, those that live in the blood and those that live in the intestines, and the former are the ones that cause serious diseases, though fortunately they are limited in distribution. Only one of these diseases, dourine (discussed elsewhere in this volume), occurs in the United States. Other dangerous protozoan diseases not occurring in the United States are surra, carried by horseflies; nagana (African sleeping sickness), carried by the tsetse fly; mal de caderas, probably carried by horseflies and stableflies; murrina, carried by vampire bats; and piroplasmosis, carried by ticks.

About 50 species of ciliated protozoa–those equipped with hair-like organs for moving around-live in the intestines, but there is no evidence that they cause disease; in fact, some of them may be useful. There are also several other protozoa, about which little is known, in various parts of the body.

The worm parasites are much more important economically than the protozoa, but the harm they do is insidious, general, and often hard to diagnose.

The strongyles are perhaps the most important single group of worms; there are about 40 species all told, of two different types, large and small, but only about 15 species are really significant. An infestation of 30 to 50 thousand strongyles in an animal is considered moderate; when the number goes over 50 thousand, relatively severe symptoms are likely to result, including lack of appetite, anemia, and progressive emaciation. The strongyles live in various parts of the large bowel. The females lay eggs, which pass out with the manure and develop into infective larvae. Animals swallow these larvae while grazing. The bloodsucking worms cause anemia, internal hemorrhages, colic, and stoppage of blood vessels, which may result in intermittent lameness.

At least eight other kinds of worm parasites besides the strongyles are harmful to horses and mules.

(1) Flukes sometimes attack the liver, blood vessels, and alimentary tract, but they are not normal parasites of equines.

(2) Three species of tapeworms are important economically–a large one that causes intestinal catarrh; a smaller one that commonly causes an intestinal obstruction, which may be fatal; and a dwarf tapeworm, less damaging than the other two.

(3) Four species of stomach worms cause a serious inflammation of the stomach called verminous gastritis. Three of these worms are transmitted by stableflies and horseflies. The larvae of some of the stomach worms also cause the skin disease known as summer sores, or bursati. Infestation with the small stomach worm is considered to be the most common forerunner of a sudden loss of condition in horses.

(4) The ascarids, or large roundworms, are particularly dangerous to foals and young animals. The larvae migrate through the liver and lungs, often causing extensive damage, and eventually reach the small intestine, which may become completely obstructed.

(5) The small, slender worms called *Strongyloides* infect the small intestine of nursing foals and are probably partly responsible for cases of scours.

(6) Pinworms live in the large intestine, and the females crawl out of the anal opening and rupture, leaving deposits of eggs and causing intense irritation, evidenced by tail rubbing.

(7) Lungworms, which reach the lungs after extensive migrations in the body, cause a chronic cough and bronchitis in heavy infestations.

(8) Two species of threadworms (filarire), probably transmitted by insects, infest horses. One, seldom serious, causes an inflammation and discharge of fluid into the body cavity. The other attacks a ligament in the neck and probably plays an important part in the development of poll evil, or fistulous withers.

Foster discusses various remedies used in the treatment of some of the protozoan diseases, including antimony and arsenic compounds injected into the veins.

Among the anthelmintics, or worm medicines, carbon disulfide is commonly used for roundworms. The remedies for strongyles include oil of chenopodium, carbon tetrachloride, normal butylidene chloride, and normal butyl chloride. Each of these drugs has certain serious effects on the animal, and all should be administered only with expert knowledge and care. The new anthelmintic, phenothiazine, developed by the Bureau of Animal Industry, is free of most of the drawbacks of the other drugs and can be administered in anyone of several different ways. Occasionally, however, phenothiazine produces intoxication which may lead to death.

As for prevention–the author emphasizes the need for cleanliness and good sanitation around stables and barns, and for maintaining good pastures, not overstocked. The best way to combat parasites is to pay attention to these details and give the animals periodic medication.

Mange of Equines

Mange, scabies, scab, or itch in equines is caused, as in other animals, by three species of mites, the sarcoptic, psoroptic, and chorioptic, described by Imes. Usually the disease is transmitted by direct contact, but it may be carried in other ways, since both the mites and the eggs can live for a time off the host animals; hence when mange appears, the premises and equipment should be cleaned and disinfected, and all the horses should be treated.

Itching and the formation of blisterlike vesicles and of scabs are characteristic signs of mange, but a definite diagnosis must be based on, finding the mites. Sarcoptic mites penetrate the upper layer of skill and make burrows in which mating and egg-laying take place. Psoroptic and chorioptic mites live on the surface of the skin, the latter being confined mainly to the lower parts of the legs and to the tail.

Treatment for mange consists in dipping the animals in a vat containing, usually, either a lime-sulfur or a nicotine solution. For the psoroptic and chorioptic types, two dippings are made 10 to 12 days apart, since the first does not kill the eggs and it is necessary to wait until the next generation of mites hatches. For sarcoptic mites four or more dippings, 6 or 7 days apart, may be required. The mites, buried in their tunnels, are hard to reach, and old chronic cases may be practically incurable. When there are only a few horses to be treated, the solution may be applied with a spray pump instead of in the form of a dip.

Horse Bots and Their Control

Horse botflies specialize in attacking animals of the horse family, though occasionally a young larva, or bot, burrows into the skill of a human being. Three of the four species of these flies are common in the United States. As Bishopp and Schwartz make clear, each has its own fiendishly ingenious way of getting its larvae inside the bodies of horses.

The nose botfly hovers about the head of a horse and suddenly darts in to attach its eggs, one at a time, to hairs on the lips. When the eggs hatch, the young bots burrow for a month or so in the mucous membrane lining the mouth. They then pass to the stomach and intestines, where they remain 8 to 11 months, perforating the lining membranes and causing considerable damage in addition to paving the way for germ infections. Finally, grown to full size, they pass to the rectum and thence leave the animal. On or in the ground, the larvae become pupae and then develop into flies.

The throat botfly attaches its eggs to hairs not on the lips but under the jaw. The young larvae crawl into the mouth and establish themselves in pockets in the gums, between the molars. Then they too pass to the stomach and intestines.

The common horse botfly attaches its eggs to hairs on the horse's body and legs, usually on the inner side of the knee. These eggs will not hatch until the horse bites and rubs the infested spot. Then, stimulated by the warmth and rubbing, the larvae burst the eggs open, stick to the horse's lips, burrow into the mucous membranes of the lips and tongue, and ultimately pass to the stomach and intestines.

The attacks of nose and throat botflies, especially the former, are maddening to horses, and they do everything they can to escape the creatures.

The adult flies cannot eat, and the females are simply egg-laying machines; hence they cannot be attracted to traps or poisoned bait.

Nor is there any practical way of killing the eggs. Three methods of control are use, however.

(1) As a protection against the attacks of the nose botfly, fasten a broad band, 4 to 6 inches wide, beneath the lips, attaching the ends to the bit rings. A piece of burlap hung under the jaw will similarly keep off the throat botfly. Unfortunately these simple devices cannot be used readily while the animals are grazing.

(2) After heavy freezes have killed all common botflies, rub the infested parts of the horse's legs with a swab or sponge soaked with warm water (105° to 110°F.). This causes many of the eggs to hatch, and the exposed larvae soon die.

(3) To destroy the bots in the stomach, use carbon disulfide as a worm medicine; preferably a single dose administered in gelatin capsules or by a stomach tube (1.5 fluid drams, or 6 cubic centimeters, for each 250 pounds of body weight–6 drams for a 1,000-pound horse). A veterinarian should do the dosing, and it should be done early in the winter–December or January, depending on the locality. Cooperative community campaigns in which all the horses in an area are rounded up and treated at one time by the local veterinarians have proved to be very successful.

Some Insect Pests of Horses and Mules

In this article Bishopp gives much information in little space on a number of insects that for the most part are not discussed elsewhere in this volume.

Mosquitoes and sand flies (punkies)–Often very annoying to animals. Mosquitoes can carry encephalomyelitis, or sleeping sickness. Control measures include screening, use of pyrethrum sprays, eliminating stagnant water, using oil on pools, pasturing livestock on high ground, using smudges.

Houseflies–Annoy animals; transmit some parasites and diseases. Control measures include proper disposal and handling of manure and vegetable refuse, screening, use of fly traps and pyrethrum sprays.

Horseflies and deer flies–Bloodsucking; bites are painful; carry some very serious diseases. Control, which is difficult, involves eliminating breeding places (swamps, marshes, etc.) Darkened sheds and smudges give some protection.

Buffalo gnats (blackfles)–Severe outbreaks greatly affect the condition of animals; may be fatal. The gnats breed in running water, and control is difficult. Bishopp discusses special handling of streams, use of poison in streams, pasturing on high ground, use of repellants, inoculation with gnat extract.

Fleas–Discussed elsewhere in this volume.

Lice–Three kinds are found on equines. Control is by application of suitable insecticides, especially by dipping.

Ticks–Several kinds attack equines. Treatment with a pine tarcottonseed oil mixture is used for those that attack the ears; arsenical dips, or washing or dusting with rotenone mixtures, are advised for those that attack the body.

Chapter 1

EQUINE ENCEPHALOMYELITIS

L.T. Giltner and M.S. Shahan[1]

[1] *L.T. Giltner is Senior Veterinarian and M.S. Shahan is Veterinarian, Pathological Division, Bureau of Animal Industry.*

The Same Virus that causes encephalomyelitis in horses can also cause sleeping sickness (encephalitis) in human beings. Both maladies belong in a group of serious diseases of the central nervous system that includes poliomyelitis (infantile paralysis) of human beings. The intensive research work on encephalomyelitis in recent years is both significant and unusually interesting.

It is estimated that since 1930 nearly a million horses and mules in the United States have been affected by infectious encephalomyelitis. The disease, known popularly as sleeping sickness and brain fever, is believed to have been present in this country for several decades, although the specific cause–a filterable virus–was not discovered here until 1930 (*40*).[2]

In 1930 and 1931, an estimated 6,000 horses and mules contracted the disease in California alone (*39*). During the next few years the malady gradually spread eastward through Arizona, Oregon, South Dakota, Colorado, and Nebraska, finally involving every section and practically every State in this country and some of the Canadian Provinces.

---

[2] Italic number in parenthesis refer to literature cited.

In 1933 the disease appeared along the Atlantic seaboard, in Delaware, Maryland, New Jersey, and Virginia. From these cases a type of virus different from that found in the West was identified (*41, 21, 57, 67*).This so-called eastern type of virus was found to be more deadly than the western type, and in addition it was determined that recovery from infection with one type did not immunize an animal against the other. The two types are thus what is known as immunologically distinct, even though both produce essentially the same clinical disease. During the years 1939 to 1941 the western type of the disease spread from California to Kentucky and Alabama, being especially prevalent in the watershed of the Mississippi River. The eastern type in the same period spread chiefly along the Atlantic coast into Florida, Georgia, Massachusetts, North Carolina, and South, Carolina, Inland into Alabama, and along the Gulf coast to Mexico (*46, 71*). So far as is known, the two types of virus have up to the time of writing remained geographically separated, except in Alabama (*59*) and Texas (*46, 71*).

Symptoms

There are certain indications of infectious equine encephalomyelitis and clinically similar diseases that should be known by everyone handling horses, mules, asses. Nearly every animal that has sleeping sickness develops fever, sleepiness, grinding of the teeth, wobbly gait, and more or less difficulty in chewing and swallowing.

The first indication, fever, is present in practically all cases. The temperature varies from 102° to 107° F. During the early part of the febrile stage, nothing more indicative of illness than lack of spirit or slightly peculiar actions may be noticed, but it is at this time especially that the virus of the disease is present in the blood (*19, 48 56*) and multiplying rapidly. The disease may then terminate, if the infection is of the so-called inapparent or occult type; or it may progress, causing distinct symptoms of involvement of the central nervous system (brain and spinal cord) and constituting what is known as the frank case. Both types of attack constitute true infections, and a considerable degree of immunity results from either. These observations have been made in both experimental and field cases (*15, 66*). It is believed that during an outbreak many animals, interspersed among the frank cases and the apparently wholly normal animals, develop occult infections. In an epizootic area during an outbreak, animals with this type of the disease may be found in almost any stable.

Sluggishness and drowsiness are early symptoms in the developing case of infectious equine encephalomyelitis. The lips become loose and droopy or are tensed and wrinkled or drawn to one side. Groups of muscles about the head, shoulder, or flank may be seen to twitch spasmodically. With the progress of the disease, the animal stands dejctedly and moves reluctantly with an awkward stumbling or staggering gait (Fig. 1). Some affected, animals are inclined to back persistently or walk stumblingly in a circle in one direction, the tail switching as they move. Such animals may blunder blindly into obstructions in their path. Whinnying is a common symptom. In many cases there is extreme sensitiveness, as shown by flinching at the slightest touch or by jerking muscular contractions when the animal is excited by unusual sounds. In most cases the animals are stupid and intractable, but a few become wild and unmanageable as in furious rabies. Sometimes sexual excitement occurs.

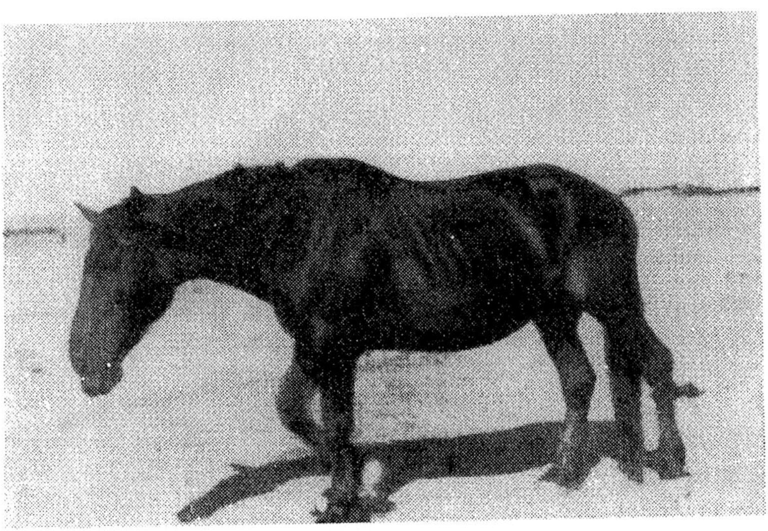

Fig. 1: A horse with a typical case of sleeping sickness. (Courtesy of Veterinary Science Division, University of California).

The dejected "sleeper" when aroused may exhibit momentary interest in feed or water, only soon to lapse into a stupor with unchewed food in the mouth or water trickling from the lips or nostrils. The lips, tongue, or cheeks may be paralyzed, but in most cases the difficulty in swallowing appears to come from inability to coordinate the normal muscular activity; often if the water bucket is held up to the animal and he is repeatedly aroused, he may succeed in obtaining a considerable quantity of water, a small amount at a time.

During the periods of stupor, grinding of the teeth is common. Stretching of the neck and head in a yawning motion is frequently observed. There is usually a slight watery discharge from the nostrils, and the mouth becomes foul smelling owing to the accumulation and putrefaction of secretions and unswallowed food. If the eye is examined carefully, the membranes will invariably be found to be congested and of a dull yellowish or muddy color. Sometimes small hemorrhages are present.

With the progress of the illness, the animal becomes increasingly gaunt, and there is commonly prominent ridge due to muscular tenseness along the lower abdominal wall. The digestive and excretory processes are retarded, and more or less constipation or sluggishness of the bowels results. Urine collects in the bladder, which may become greatly distended. Dribbling of urine without normal periodic voiding is common.

In about 1 of every 4 or 5 cases due to the western type of virus and 9 of every 10 cases caused by the eastern type, the animal gradually becomes weaker and weaker, finally collapsing on the ground. Very few of those that go down and are unable to regain their feet unaided recover, though it may be hours or days before the end. During this time they may lie quietly, breathing with a snoring sound, or they may thrash about considerably. Some animals literally bury themselves, digging up the earth with running movements of the legs in their delirium. Marked bruising and swelling develop on the parts of the body in contact with the ground.

If the animal lies quietly, the body temperature is usually normal or only slightly raised at this stage, but if there is much struggling or if complications such as pneumonia or other organic diseases occur there may be considerable fever. Among the animals that survive a typical attack of the disease, a few–the so-called dummies–retain evidence of more or less permanent injury to the brain and spinal cord.[3]

Development and Spread of the Disease

Infectious equine encephalomyelitis is essentially an epizootic disease–that is, one occurring in outbreaks that correspond to epidemics among human beings. While scattered or sporadic cases may occur at any time during the warm months, the peak of an epizootic is usually reached during July, August, or September in most sections. The disease invariably disappears after the first sharp frosts of fall. There is only one proved winter case on record, and that occurred in Florida in January during a mild season (*43*).

Sleeping sickness is essentially a disease of pastured animals, occurring only rarely among those continuously stabled. This is considered to be one of the reasons why Army posts and Thoroughbred breeding establishments remain relatively free from it.

The malady strikes hardest in farm and ranch areas along or near a stream, lake, marsh, swamp, or the seashore. In the West, irrigated sections are especially affected, as well as arid regions when unusually heavy rains occur. In the East, the tidewater regions have the most cases. Scattered or sporadic cases may be observed early in the summer and throughout the warm months under conditions of drought. On the other hand, heavy rains that result in the flooding of pastures and waste land and the formation of pools are frequently followed in 2 or 3 weeks by large numbers of cases. Under the latter conditions, extended hot weather also appears to be a factor in promoting the spread of the disease. Both moisture and heat, of course, encourage the breeding and feeding activities of insects.

There is a tendency for the disease to occur sporadically for one or more seasons in a given locality and then, under conditions favorable to it, to become very severe and widespread for one or more seasons. Following a severe and extended epizootic period, the disease may practically or entirely disappear for several years, only to reassert itself later when circumstances again become favorable.

---

[3] Detailed clinical descriptions of the disease are presented in citations, 6, 10, 17, 39, 49.

During severe outbreaks, 10 percent or more of the horses and mules in an area may show unmistakable signs of the sickness. It is seldom that more than one or a few of the animals on a given farm sicken. Cases are often separated by several miles, and some premises appear to escape altogether. However, the virus probably attacks more animals than is superficially apparent, producing occult infections.

The incubation period of the naturally acquired disease (the time elapsing between entrance of the virus into the body and the appearance of the first symptoms) is believed to vary in length, as does this period in artificially infected animals. In the latter, the first symptoms usually appear 3 to 10 days after the introduction of the virus, depending on the dose and route of injection and on the type of virus. In some unusual cases as long as 3 weeks may elapse.

Although it is generally believed that horses of all ages and breeds are susceptible. there is some evidence to indicate that certain breeds may be less resistant than others (*30*). Certainly animals that have been exposed to the infection through the course of one or more outbreaks may be reasonably assumed to be more resistant as a class than others; such as colts, which have never before encountered the disease. Heredity, age, and nutrition are all suspected of playing a part in the artificially produced disease in mice, and these may be factors in the case of horses also.

Tests with guinea pigs indicate that young animals nursing immune mothers are highly resistant to the disease (*20*). Foals and young horses are believed to be more likely to recover than older horses. There is a widespread opinion among practicing veterinarians, to some extent supported by available data, that mules are less susceptible than horses (*51*).

It is generally believed that the disease is transmitted by bloodsucking insects. It has been found experimentally that at least 11 species of mosquitoes, all of the genus *Aedes*, can be infected, and 10 of these are capable of transmitting the virus (*9, 16, 26, 27, 33, 34, 36, 61*). Some species have been found that are practically incapable of transmitting one type of virus but that infect with the other type with a single bite (*15, 37*). Other species transmit both types with equal facility. Some of these mosquitoes are known to be widely distributed in the United States, others are somewhat restricted in distribution; but all except one species are present to some extent in one or more of the sections where the disease has occurred (*5*). Mosquitoes (*Culex tarsalis*) naturally infected with the western type of virus were discovered in the Yakima Valley, Wash., in 1941 (*16*). Numerous fruitless attempts had been made to find the virus in mosquitoes and other insects (including horseflies, houseflies, stableflies, hornflies, and spinose ear ticks) in nature (*44, 56, 70*) before this important finding was reported.

The virus has been reported as present in so-called assassin bugs (*Triatoma sanguisuga*) (*29*) collected in Kansas where the disease has been prevalent. This bug is relatively infrequently found in comparison with other insects that might be suspected as vectors (carriers) and probably cannot be held solely responsible for the dissemination of the equine disease. The chief importance of finding infection in this species would seem to lie in the probable existence of a reservoir for the virus somewhere among the many kinds of victims of its bite.

The tick that transmits Rocky Mountain spotted fever (*Dermacentor andersoni*) has been found to be capable of transmitting equine encephalomyelitis virus under experimental conditions (*63*). Moreover, it has been shown to transmit the virus from one generation to the next through the eggs and larvae (*64*). Like other ticks, these are relatively long-lived, and it is easy to conceive of their carrying the virus through the winter, or even through several years, and then transmitting it to susceptible species for further propagation, as has been suggested (*62*). The fact that the disease can readily be transmitted under certain conditions by several species of arthropods, particularly mosquitoes, must be accepted. However, that they actually do transmit it under natural conditions, or that they are the sole means of transmission, remains unproved despite very strong circumstantial evidence supporting the theory.

What becomes of the virus with the seasonal subsidence of the disease in horses is unknown. No evidence has yet been presented which proves that horses harbor the virus from one epizootic season to the next. Inasmuch as the virus is capable of surviving for only a relatively short time outside the animal body, it is assumed that it is perpetuated in some species other than the horse, mule, or ass.

Man was suspected as early as 1932 of being susceptible to the virus of sleeping sickness of American horses (*38*), and the possibility that he might act as a reservoir of the virus was considered in 1935

(*66*). The eastern type of equine virus was first actually demonstrated in cases of disease of the brain in man in 1938 (*12, 72*). Other cases, some due to the western type of virus, were subsequently identified (*11, 32*), and it is now an accepted fact that man is susceptible to the disease, which, as far as is known at present, is not immunologically related to the somewhat similar diseases, infantile paralysis (poliomyelitis) and epidemic encephalitis (St. Louis type). In many if not most cases of the equine virus disease in human beings there has been no evidence of contact with horses, and it is assumed that people generally contract the infection from the same source as horses, though a few cases have occurred among laboratory workers and some among persons closely associated with sick horses. Children have been especially affected in some outbreaks. The virus recovered from the brain of a child has produced typical equine encephalomyelitis when injected into susceptible horses. Encephalitis in man due to the equine virus is a very serious disease at any age, but there is a particularly high mortality rate among children affected with the eastern type, and troublesome complications are reported to be common in those surviving. The disease caused by the western type of virus is relatively much less severe than that due to the eastern type. On the other hand, the former has been more widespread. Over 2,000 cases, mostly attributed to the equine virus (western type), were reported from North Dakota, South Dakota, Minnesota, Montana, and Nebraska in 1941.

It has been determined that horses are susceptible to human encephalitis (St. Louis type) virus when artificially inoculated, and in areas where sleeping sickness has been epizootic in horses, people and animals have been found the serum from which was capable of neutralizing the virus of that disease as well as the virus of infectious equine encephalomyelitis (*8, 23, 24, 45*). The assumption is that both viruses may produce the disease in horses and other animals as well as in man and that the two have existed simultaneously in some outbreaks of both the human and the equine disease, although St. Louis encephalitis virus has never been found naturally occurring in equines. The viruses of St. Louis encephalitis and equine encephalomyelitis have both been found in mosquitoes (*Culex tarsalis*) (*16*).

A disease of the central nervous system due to equine encephalomyelitis virus has been found to occur naturally in ring-necked pheasants, pigeons, and prairie chickens (*3, 7*). Thus, it is definitely known that birds are sometimes attacked by the virus of so-called brain fever of horses. This disease has no known connection with the virus disease of chickens known as chick encephalomyelitis or epidemic tremors (*42*).

A disease in ducks in Montana suspected of being encephalomyelitis was investigated in 1938, but the presence of the equine virus was not actually demonstrated (*60*). This outbreak, as well as the proved cases in pigeons, pheasants, and prairie chickens, occurred in an area where sleeping sickness of horses had been prevalent.

It is now known that over 20 species of birds are susceptible to the virus of sleeping sickness when artificially injected. Following inoculation by certain methods, hens and turkeys have been found to develop transitory in apparent infections with virus circulating in the blood stream (*65*). A similar condition has been shown with certain species of blackbirds and the mourning dove, cowbird, and grackle (*9*). Such birds, without showing obvious indications of infection, may play roles in the spread of the disease as important as or even more important than those of others which, like pigeons and pheasants, develop frank symptoms of encephalomyelitis and have a high death rate from the disease. The list of susceptible birds includes ducks, geese, a species of hawk, blackbirds, the tawny vulture, the white stork, guinea fowl, English sparrow, Gambel sparrow, quail, LeConte thrasher, the junco, the western burrowing owl, the American egret, red-shafted flicker, killdeer, and robin, besides those already mentioned.

Equine encephalomyelitis virus when artificially injected is capable of infecting more species of animals than perhaps any other known virus. About as many species of mammals as of birds have been so infected. In addition to the commonly used laboratory mammals–guinea pigs, white mice, white rats, rabbits and monkeys–cattle, swine, sheep, goats, dogs, cats, several species of wild mice, rats, and other rodents including rabbits, gophers, hedgehogs, and woodchucks may be infected. The list also includes weasels, ferrets, and hamsters (ratlike rodents of eastern Europe). Some species appear to be susceptible to both types of virus, while some can be infected with one type but not the other.

Although horses,. mules, and human beings are the only mammalian species now known to contract the disease naturally, many others equally susceptible to artificial exposure may eventually be found naturally affected. In fact, the virus has recently been isolated from a wild deer in Montana. The studies being made by several agencies will probably lead to the identification of other naturally infected animals and eventually to important biological reservoirs of the virus.

While it is possible that horses may occasionally contract the disease by inhaling or swallowing virus from affected animals, judging from the observed facts, transmission by such means must be exceedingly rare. Several deliberate attempts to induce the disease in normal horses by putting them in contact with affected horses have failed (*68, 69*). In fact, in all the literature on the disease not one proved instance is mentioned of infection of normal animals by contact with infected animals of any species or with an environment that might have been contaminated. The tentative conclusion, based on the available information, that the disease is chiefly arthropod-borne, is inescapable, although more work remains to be done to prove it.

Diagnosis

The diagnosis of infectious equine encephalomyelitis is based on a study of the symptoms in each case and such features as seasonal occurrence and distribution in the locality. However, because atypical cases do occur and unusual conditions are not infrequently encountered, a specific laboratory diagnosis (*59*) may be required for confirmation of clinical diagnosis or the determination of the type of virus involved.

If virus is sought in the living animal, repeated samplings of the blood very early in the course of the ailment, preferably before symptoms of disease of the nervous system appear, are usually required. The virus is present in the blood stream for only a comparatively short time and then becomes fixed in the brain and spinal cord, only rarely being found elsewhere after that. It is shown to be present by the inoculation of the finely emulsified nervous tissue from the suspected case into any of the available susceptible animals, usually guinea pigs or white mice; or the tissue may be inoculated into hen's eggs containing 9- to 13-day-old living embryos. Symptoms like those seen in horses develop in the guinea pig or mouse in a few days, and death usually results. The inoculated embryo succumbs to the virus in 15 to 24 hours (*18*). The virus is similarly demonstrable in the body of the inoculated animal and in the embryo, and it may be transmitted by inoculation from the original guinea pig, mouse, or embryo to others in long, continuous series.

If a horse or mule has been dead for some time or even prostrate for several days, it may be impossible to demonstrate virus in the tissue of the central nervous system. A few known artificially produced cases also fail to yield virus. It is then necessary to resort to microscopic examination of the tissues (*4, 25, 28, 31*). In the brain and spinal cord, the blood vessels are found to be engorged or swollen, and small hemorrhages, edema, and abnormal accumulations of various types of cells in the spaces surrounding the blood vessels or in other parts of the tissues are present. Varying degrees of degeneration of the nerve cells are to be observed. Somewhat similar but less characteristic changes may be found in the liver.

These changes are not apparent to the naked eye, although very minute hemorrhagic points may be seen in certain parts of the brain. The cerebrospinal fluid (surrounding the brain and spinal cord) is clear but greatly increased in amount and chemically and microscopically abnormal. The throat and nasal passages may be inflamed, and a putrid odor may be present. Usually the lungs are essentially normal, although there may be congestion or even pneumonia, especially in animals that have been down for some time. The stomach usually contains a considerable amount of watery, foul-smelling food material. Evidence of catarrhal inflammation and sluggishness of the bowels are common. The bladder is usually distended with clear, amber-colored, sirupy urine. The liver, instead of being slate-colored as normally, is slightly enlarged and of a dull, yellowish-gray color. The various membranes of the body also are usually dull yellowish, owing to staining with bile. The muscles appear dry and lighter colored than normal as a result of great loss of water (dehydration) by the sick animal. These changes are not necessarily characteristic of sleeping sickness, and unqualified diagnosis of the disease by this means alone is rarely if ever justified, but a thorough post mortem examination is nevertheless often a great assistance to the veterinarian in identifying other diseases that may be responsible in suspected cases.

Experimental studies have been made of the complement-fixation test (involving the use of blood serum, virus, and red blood cells) as applied to sleeping sickness, but it has not yet been generally used in diagnosis (*22, 41*). The blood serum of a convalescing or recovered animal may be tested to determine its power to inactivate or neutralize encephalomyelitis virus (in vitro neutralization test) (*14, 15, 19, 38, 66, 67*). A positive reaction to this test is generally accepted as evidence of past or present infection, the neutralizing substances constituting a form of antibody.

Similar Disease and Conditions

Not all cases of illness in horses and mules in which there is evidence of disturbance of the central nervous system are infectious encephalomyelitis.

Toxic encephalitis, as contrasted with infectious encephalomyelitis, may occur at any time of the year–in the dead of winter as well as in midsummer. However, the commonest form, that known as moldy corn poisoning (*55*), usually makes its appearance in the late fall or the winter in horses or mules that have been fed on moldy, stunted, or otherwise deteriorated or inferior corn. This malady has been responsible for the death of thousands of valuable horses from time to time in several of the Corn Belt States, usually in the months of November to April after an unusually dry summer and heavy fall rains.

The symptoms of moldy corn poisoning are scarcely distinguishable from those of other clinically similar ailments by any but the trained observer. Usually, however, there is no yellowness of the membranes of the body and no great rise in body temperature. At autopsy, areas of softening and degeneration sometimes microscopic only but more often plainly evident to the naked eye, are usually found in the brain.

Prevention consists in avoiding the feeding of corn or corn fodder about the absolute soundness of which there is the slightest doubt. Other species of animals may tolerate poor corn, but is dangerous to horses in this and other ways. It may be desirable in some instances to muzzle horses being worked in the corn harvest in order to prevent their eating potentially dangerous corn. Although moldiness is considered as an important indication of danger, unfortunately it is not always possible to determine by examination whether a certain lot of corn can be fed with safety. The toxin in bad corn, whatever its nature, appears to be cumulative in effect, and symptoms do not ordinarily develop in less than a month, even though the corn is fed continuously.

There is no specific remedy for the disease, and the medicinal aid given by the veterinarian varies somewhat with the conditions found in each case.

Other toxins or poisons in some deteriorated feeds other than corn, as well as some mineral poisons such as barium, lead, arsenic, phosphorus, and selenium, may cause symptoms attributable to or suggestive of encephalitis. Among the plants that may induce more or less similar symptoms are whorled milkweed, yellow tarweed, poisonhemlock, ragwort, locoweed, ergot-infested paspalum grass, and horsetail. Unripe and green as well as rotten or sprouted potatoes are very dangerous feed for horses or other animals and often produce symptoms suggestive of encephalitis. Certain ticks engorging on various animals, including the horse, sometimes cause a peculiar form of paralysis, which is usually promptly remedied by the removal of the ticks.

Such diseases as anthrax and influenza (shipping fever) sometimes cause encephalitis. Some cases of acute infectious anemia (swamp fever) show symptoms that resemble those of infectious encephalomyelitis. Rabies, a virus disease transmitted by the bite of an infected animal, usually a dog, is a form of encephalitis. Still other infectious diseases may cause symptoms of nervous disease. Even tetanus, or lockjaw, has been diagnosed as infectious encephalomyelitis by untrained persons. Diagnosis and treatment vary according to the nature of the primary disease in question.

Some animals affected by heat stroke or lightning develop spasms, convulsions, or residual paralysis, which must be differentiated from true encephalitis. These, of course, are usually isolated cases.

Tumors of various types and abscesses in the brain arising from bacterial infection may cause symptoms suggesting infectious encephalomyelitis. Close clinical examination and a study of the history of these comparatively rare cases will usually enable the experienced veterinarian to identify the condition. The same may be said of mechanical injuries to the head.

Botulism (*13*) is a disease caused by the ingestion of a toxin produced in feeds under certain conditions by a widely distributed germ known as *Clostridium botulinum*. The chief symptom consists of progressive paralysis, usually beginning in the eyes, tongue, and throat, finally involving the entire body, and resulting in death.

Azoturia, sometimes referred to as Monday morning disease because it commonly occurs in well-fed and under-exercised horses after a week end of rest in the stable, has been confused with infectious encephalomyelitis.

In the last decade, in several States in areas where infectious encephalomyelitis had previously prevailed, a second illness, now called toxic hepatogenous icterus,[4] in some ways resembling sleeping sickness and in others quite different, has appeared during the late fall and early winter 2 weeks to 2 months after epizootics of sleeping sickness (*35, 58*). Usually horses affected with this disease have no fever, develop an obstinate constipation and extreme icterus (jaundice), and become very unmanageable, pushing violently against any objects in their path. The affection is extremely acute and the death rate high. Studies conducted to date do not prove that it is infectious, and its true nature is not yet definitely known. Although many of the animals that have developed this affiction had been treated earlier with anti-encephalomyelitis serum, some had not.

The chief abnormality found at autopsy is a damaged liver, which shows characteristic changes under the microscope. Success in treatment appears to depend chiefly on early diagnosis and prompt stimulation of the intestinal tract.

Control and Prevention

Although not everything is known about the spread of sleeping sickness, as has been pointed out, nevertheless there are certain justifiable, practical, and apparently effective means of prevention. The selection and application of these measures, singly or collectively, must properly be considered as technical matters. Accordingly, when control of the disease is to be attempted, a licensed veterinary practitioner or authorized veterinary official should be

---

[4] The term "toxic hepatogenous icterus" has been proposed to replace the previously used terms "secondary disease" or "X disease." See MOHLER, J.R. REPORT ON INFECTIOUS EQUINE ENCEPHALOMYELITIS IN THE UNITED STATES IN 1939. U.S. Bur. Anim. Indus., 5 pp., illus. 1940. (Mimeographed.)

consulted. In the past, much money has been spent needlessly by frantic horse owners for worthless and in some cases even harmful so-called preventives or cures for infectious encephalomyelitis.

(1) Among the means of prevention, vaccination is of first importance. The approved, commercially available vaccine of today consists of artificially infected chick-embryo tissue, in which the power of the virus to produce the disease has been destroyed by the addition of a solution of formaldehyde (2). Other products have been tried with more of less success, but all have been displaced by the present one of chick-embryo origin known as encephalomyelitis vaccine. The vaccine is prepared from embryos infected with western, eastern, or both types of virus. Which should be used depends upon the type of virus known to prevail in the locality.

Since the virus is rendered harmless by the presence of formaldehyde in the vaccine, there is no danger of producing the disease in animals injected with the product. It is thus unlike some other products used for the control of animal diseases, but it is not so foolproof that it can be safely and effectively used by everyone. Its proper administration requires the services of a veterinarian who understands that the product deteriorates and becomes less effective, if not worthless, when not properly handled. Then, too, severe reactions and even death have been known to occur following vaccination (*52, 53*). These undesirable results can be largely if not wholly prevented by injecting the vaccine into the skin (*54*) rather than under it or into the muscles, as was once practiced.

While one dose of the vaccine results in an appreciable degree of resistance, it lasts for only a comparatively short time. Accordingly two doses at 7- to 10-day intervals should be given. Unfortunately many farmers do not have their animals vaccinated until the disease has already made its appearance on their farms or in their vicinity, and under these conditions the method is not fully effective. Although vaccination during an outbreak appears to be safe and effective as: a last resort, such a procedure cannot be expected to be as advantageous as vaccination before the epizootic season, which extends from July to October in most sections but is somewhat earlier in others. To secure the maximum protection during these months, the, two-dose vaccination should preferably be completed not later than early July in most localities. In some areas vaccination in the early spring or even late winter may be advisable. Experimental tests indicate that most vaccinated animals develop immunity within 10 days to 2 weeks after the administration of the second dose of vaccine and retain a sufficient degree of immunity to resist even the severest artificial exposure for 6 months and sometimes even longer (*50, 60*). In order to assure protection, it appears at present that animals should be revaccinated each year.

(2) Second among preventive procedures is the prevention or limitation of bites by bloodsucking insects, particularly mosquitoes. Prevention or control of breeding of the insects, screening of stables, stabling of horses and mules as much as possible, the use of nets, etc., on working animals, and the frequent application to the animals and the premises of repellent compounds are all useful.

(3) All animals affected with the disease should be stabled in screened quarters or kept thoroughly sprayed with an effective repellent, especially in the early stage of the disease when the blood is infectious. If possible, a separate caretaker should be provided for them. Although it is probable that man does not contract the disease from horses or other affected animals by direct contact, those engaged in handling or treating such animals should avoid unnecessary risks, especially from soiling the hands or person with secretions or excretions from the sick animals.

(4) Extermination of rats, mice, and other vermin and exclusion from the places where the horses are kept of pigeons and stray or wild animals are advisable on general principles.

(5) Although rigid general quarantine measures have not been found practical in dealing with encephalomyelitis, the movement of horses or mules from an epizootic area into a clean area should be discouraged. When it is necessary, the animals might well be vaccinated at least 15 days before being moved. Animals going into an infected area from one

where the disease has not been prevalent should be similarly treated.

(6) Animals dead of the disease should be promptly disposed of by thorough rendering or burning or deep burial with the addition of quick time. The stables, sheds, corrals, etc., used by the affected animals should be thoroughly cleaned, and feed boxes, stalls, watering troughs, etc., should be disinfected with either a 2-percent aqueous solution of lye or a 1-percent solution of formalin. The formalin will in time evaporate from the treated surfaces, but lye should be thoroughly removed after a few hours by repeated washing with clean water.

(7) A specific anti-encephalomyelitis serum (*19, 20, 38, 47*) is commercially available, and some experimental data indicate that it has some preventive value. Practical considerations, however, considerably restrict its use in the prevention of the disease, and vaccine is preferred in most instances.

Vaccination properly done does not interfere with working or breeding the animals. A few instances of abortion have been reported in pregnant mares vaccinated by the older method, but none following intradermic vaccination. A small, hard swelling may remain at the site of injection for as long as a few weeks, but this does no harm unless it is situated where harness or saddle will rub it, and it is eventually completely resorbed.

Laboratory workers exposed to unusual danger of contracting the infection have been safely vaccinated with a product of the same general type as that used for horses (*1*), but it has not been generally used in epidemic areas.

Treatment

If despite well-advised and diligently applied control measures, sleeping sickness or anything resembling it develops in a stable, a veterinarian should be called immediately. Except for anti-encephalomyelitis serum, which if used at all must be given very early in the course of the disease and in large, frequently repeated doses, there is no specific treatment. Whether or not serum should be used is strictly a matter for the veterinarian's decision.

Reliance must be placed chiefly on good nursing, with such additional treatment as is recommended by the veterinarian for each individual case. Quiet, cool, comfortable, well-bedded quarters and protection of the animal from the sun and from self-injury are advisable.

If the animal has difficulty in standing, he may be placed in a leaning position against a padded wall or supported in a specially constructed padded frame.

Unnecessary fussing about the animal should be avoided, although almost constant attendance may be required to assist it in supporting itself. Many animals affected with sleeping sickness will not or cannot eat or drink unless the feed and water are held up to them and they are frequently aroused from their stupor. Water in small quantities, frequently given is most desirable, and if it is not or cannot be swallowed it may be given by stomach tube, by way of the rectum, or into the blood stream in the form of various solutions. Feed is not nearly so important as water. However when the animal will take small amounts of it, succulent feed may he allowed freely.

On the supposition that horses affected with encephalomyelitis, like humans with encephalitis, have a headache, cold compresses or ice packs are sometimes placed on the poll. This should do no harm and may be of benefit. Although very few animals that have been prostrate for hours or days can be expected to recover, they should be humanely treated if they are not destroyed.

Some cases may be benefited by stimulants; others may require laxatives, evacuation of the bladder by catheterization, or quieting drugs. Such drugs as are given are usually administered either through a stomach tube or hypodermically. No one system of treatment is applicable in all cases. Above all, unguided home treatment, promiscuous drenching, or other administrations which may be suggested by unqualified advisers, should not be attempted. Unwise or injudicious treatment may easily result in the needless loss of the animal. On the other hand, many horses die despite the best efforts of the most experienced and highly qualified veterinarians.

Literature Cited

(1) BEARD, J.W., BEARD, DOROTHY, and FINKELSTEIN, HAROLD (1939). HUMAN VACCINATION AGAINST EQUINE ENCEPHALOMYELITIS VIRUS WITH FORMALIZED CHICK E:MRRYO VACCINE. Science 90: 215-216.

(2) ________FINKELSTEIN, HAROLD, SEALY, W.C., and WYCKOFF, R.W.G. (1938). IMMUNIZATION AGAINST EQUINE ENCEPHALOMYELITIS WITH CHICK EMBRYO VACCINES. Science 87: 400.

(3) BEAUDETTE, F.R. (1939). EQUINE ENCEPHALOMYELITIS IN AVIAN HOSTS. U.S. Live Stock Sanit. Assoc. Proc. 43: 185-203.

(4) BIESTER, H.E., and SCHWARTE, L.H. (1936). LABORATORY CASE STUDIES OF EQUINE INCEPHALOMYELITIS. Iowa Vet. 7 (3): 13-17.

(5) BISHOPP, F.C. (1939). MOSQUITO TRANSMISSION OF ENCEPHALOMYELITIS, OR BRAIN FEVER, OF HORSES. Wash. Acad. Sci. Jour. 29: 495-501.

(6) BREUCKNER, A.L., POELMA, L.J., EVERSON, C.L., and REED, R.C. (1934). EQUINE ENCEPHALOMYELITIS. Md. Agr. Expt. Sta. Bul. 369, pp. 137-.146, illus.

(7) COX, HERALDR, JELLISON, WILLIAM L., and HUGHES, LYNDAHL E. (1941). ISOLATION OF WESTERN EQUINE ENCEPHALPHYEITIS VIRUS FROM A NATURALLY INFECTED PRAIRIE CHICKEN. U.S. Pub. Health Serv., Pub. Health Rpts. 56: 1905-1906.

(8) ________PHILLIP, CORNELIUS B., and KILPATBICK, J.W. (1941). SUSCEPTIBILITY OF HORSES TO ST. LOUIS ENOEPHALOMYELITIS VIRUS. U.S. Pub. Health Serv., Pub. Health Rpts. 56: 1391-1392.

(9) DAVIS, WILLIAM A. (1940). A SURVEY OF BIRDS AND MOSQUITOES AS HOSTS FOR THE VIRUS OF EASTERN EQUINE ENCEPHALOMYELITIS. Amer. Jour. Hyg., Protozool. and Malariol., Sect. C;32 (2): 45-59.

(10) FARQUHABSON, JAMES (1939). INFECTIOUS EQUINE ENCEPHALOMYELITIS. Amer. Vet. Med. Assoc. Jour. 94 (n.s. 47): 459-465, illus.

(11) FOTHERGILL, L[EROY] D. (1940). EQUINE ENCEPHALOMYELITIS. *In* Virus and Rickettsial Diseases With Especial Consideration of Their Public Health Significance. Harvard School of Public Health Symposium, pp. 661-683.

(12) ________DINGLE, JOHN H., and FABBER, SIDNEY (1938). HUMAN ENCEPHALITIS CAUSED BY THE VIRUS OF THE EASTERN VARIETY OF EQUINE ENCEPHALOMELITIB. New England Jour. Med. 219: (411).

(13) GEIGER, J.C., DICKSON, E.C., and MEYER, K.F. (1922). THE EPIDEMIOLOGY OF BOTULISM. U.S. Pub. Health Serv. Bul. 127, 119 pp., illus.

(14) GILTNER, L.T., and SHAHAN, M.S. (1933). THE 1933 OUTBREAK OF INFECTIOUS EQUINE ENCEPHALOMYELITIS IN THE EASTERN STATES. North Amer. Vet. 14 (11): 25-27.

(15) ________and SHAHAN, M.S. (1936). THE PRESENT STATUS OF INFECTIOUS EQUINE ENCEPHALOMYELITIS IN THE UNITED STATES. Amer. Vet. Med. Assoc. Jour. 88: 363-374.

(16) HAMMON, WILLIAM McD., REEVES, WILLIAM C., BROOKMAN, BERNARD, IZUMI, ERNEST M., and GJULLIN, C.M. (1941). ISOLATION OF THE VIRUSES OF WESTERN EQUINE AND ST. LOUIS ENCEPHALITIS FROM CULEX TARSALIS MOSQUITOES. Science 94: 828- 380.

(17) HARING, C.M., HOWARTH, J.A., and MEYER, K.F. (1931). AN INFECTIOUS BRAIN DISEASE OF HORSES AND MULES (ENCEPHALOMYELITIS.). Calif. Agr. Expt. Sta. Cir. 322, 14 pp., illus.

(18) HIGBIE, ELIZABETH, and HOWITT, BEATRICE. (1935). THE BEHAVIOR OF THE VIRUS OF EQUINE ENCEPHALOMYELITIS ON THE CHORIQALLANTOIC MEMBRANE OF THE DEVLOPING CHICK. Jour. Bact. 29: 399-400, illus.

(19) HOWITT, BFATBICE F. (1932). EQUINE ENCEPHALOMYEI.ITIS. Jour. Infect. Dis. 51: [493]-510.

(20) ________(1934). IMMUNIZATION OF GUINEA-PIGS TO THE VIRUS OF EQUINE ENCEPHAIAMYELITIS. Jour. Infect. Dis. 54: 36-87.

(21) ________(1935). AN IMMUNOLOGICAL STUDY IN LABORATORY ANIMALS OF THIBTEEN DIFFERENT STRAINS OF EQUINE ENCEPHALOMYELITIC VIBUS. Jour. Immunol. 29: 319-341.

(22) ________(1937). THE COMPLEMENT FIXATION REACTION IN EXPERIMENTAL EQUINE EN CEPHALOMYELITIS, LYMPHOCYTIC CHOMOMENINGITIS AND THE ST. LOUIS TYPE OF ENCEPHALITIS. Jour. Immunol. 33: 235-250.

(23) ________(1939). VIRUSES OF EQUINE AND OF ST. LOUIS ENCEPHALITIS IN RELATIONSHIP TO HUMAN INFECTIONS IN CALIFOBNIA, 1937-1938. Amer. Jour. Pub. Health 29: 1083-1097, illus.

(24) ________(1940). EQUINE ENCEPHALOMYELITIS; ITS RELATIONSHIP TO MAN AND ANIMALS IN CALIFORNIA. Internatl. Cong. Microbiol. Proc. 3: 302-303.

(25) HURST, E. WESTON (1934). THE HISTOLOGY OF EQUINE ENCEPHALOMYELITIS. Jour. Expt. Med. 59: 529-542, illus.

(26) KELSER, R.A. (1933). MOSQUITOES AS VECTORS OF THE VIRUS OF EQUINE ENCEPHALOMYELITIS. Amer. Vet. Med. Assoc. Jour. 82 (n.s. 35): 767-771.

(27) ________(1938). TRANSMISSION OF THE VIRUS OF EQUINE ENCEPHALOMYELITIS BY AEDES TAENIOBHYNCHUS. Amer. Vet. Med. Assoc. Jour. 92 (n.s. 45): 195-203.

(28) KING, LESTER S. (1938). STUDIES ON EASTERN EQUINE ENCEPHALOMYELITIS. I. HISTOPATHOLOGY OF THE NERVOUS SYSTEM IN THE GUINEA PIG. Jour. Expt. Med. 68: 677-691.

(29) KITSELMAN, CHARLES H., and GRUNDMANN, ALBERT W. (1940). EQUINE ENCEPHALOMYELITIS VIRUS ISOLATED FROM NATURALLY INFECTED TRIATOMA SANGUISUGA LE CONTE. Kans. Agr. Expt. Sta. Tech. Bul. 50, 15 pp., illus.

(30) LAMBERT, W.V., SPEELMAN, S R., and OSBOBN, E.B. (1939). DIFFERENCES IN INCIDENCE OF ENCEPHAI.OMYELITIBIN HORSES. Jour. Hered. 30: 349-352.

(31) LABBELL, O., HARING, C.M., and MEYER, K.F. (1934). HISTOLOGICAL CHANGES IN THE CENTRAL NERVOUS SYSTEM FOLLOWING EQUINE ENCEPHALOMYELITIS. Amer. Jour. Path. 10: 61-373.

(32) LEAKE, JAMES P. (1941). EPIDEMIC OF INFECTIOUS ENCEPHALITIS. Pub. Health Rpts. 56: 1902-1905.

(33) MADSEN, D.E. and KNOWLTON, G.F. (1935). MOSQUITO TRANSMISSION OF EQUINE ENCEPHALOMYELITIS. Med. Assoc. Jour. 6 (n.s. 39); 662-666.

(34) MADSEN, D.E., KNOWLTON,G.F., and ROWE, J.A. (1936). FURTHER STUDIES ON TRANSMISSION OF EQUINE ENCEPHALOMYELITIS BY MOSQUITOES. AMer. Vet. Med. Assoc. Jour. 89 (n.s. 42): 187-196.

(35) MARSH, HADLEIGH (1937). LOSSES OF UNDILTERMINEO CAUSE FOLLOWING AN OUTBREAK OF EQUINE ENCEPHALOMYELITIS. Amer. Vet. Med. Assoc. Jour. 91 (n.s. 44): 88-93.

(36) MERRILL, MALOOLM H., LACAILLADE, C.WM., Jr., TEN BROECK, CARL (1934). MOSQUITO TRANSMISSION OF EQUINE ENCEPHALOMYELITIS. Science 80: 251-252.

(37) ________and TEN BROECK, CABL (1935). THE TRANSMISSION OF EQUINE ENCEPHALOMYELITIS VIRUS BY AEDES AEGYPTI. Jour. Expt. Med. 62: 687-695.

(38) MEYEB, K.F. (1932). SUMMARY OF RECENT STUDIES ON. EQUINE ENCEPHALOMYELITIS. Ann. Int. Med. 6: 645-654.

(39) ________(1933). EQUINE ENCEPHALOMYELITIS. North Amer. Vet. 14 (6): 30-48.

(40) ________HARING, C.M., and HOWITT, B. (1931). THE ETIOLOGY OF EPIZOOTIC ENCEPHALOMYELITIS OF HORSES IN THE SAN JOAQUIN VALLEY, 1930. Science 74: 227-228.

(41) MOHLER, WILLIAM M. (1939). COMPLEMENT FIXATION WITH CHICK EMBRYO ANTIGEN IN EQUINE ENCEPHALOMYELITIS. Amer. Vet. Med. Assoc. Jour. 94 (n.s. 47): 39-43.

(42) OLITSKY, PETER K. (1939). EXPERIMENTAL STUDIES ON THE VIRUS OF INFECTIOUS AVIAN ENCEPHALOMYELITIS. Jour. Expt. Med. 70: 565-582, illus.

(43) OSTEEN, O.L. (1939). INFECTIOUS EQUINE ENCEPHALOMYELITIS: MID-WINTEB CASE. Amer. Vet. Med. Assoc. Jour. 94 (n.s. 47): 441-442.

(44) PHILLIP, CORNELIUS B., and COX, HERALD R. (1936). EQUINE ENCEPHALOMYELITIS IN WESTERN MONTANA IN 1936. A BRIEF DISCUSSION OF THE IMPLICATIONS OF ARTHROPOD TRANSMISSION. (Abstract) Jour. Parasitol. 22: 542.

(45) ________Cox, HERALD R., and FOUNTAIN, JOHN H. (1941). PROTECTIVE ANTIBODIES AGAINST ST. LOUIS ENCEPHALITIS VIRUS IN THE SERUM OF HORSES AND MAN. U.S. Pub. Health Serv., Pub. Health Rpts. 56: 1388-1391.

(46) RANDALL, RAYMOND, and EICHORN, ERVIN A. (1941). WEST WARD SPREAD OF EASTERN TYPE EQUINE ENCEPHALOMYELITIS VIRUS. Amer. Vet. Med. Assoc. Jour. 98: 448.

(47) RECORDS, EDWARD, and VAWTER, LYMAN R. (1933).. EQUINE ENCEPHALOMYELITIS ANTISERUM. Amer. Vet. Med. Assoc. Jour. 82 (n.s. 35): 608-616.

(48) ________and VAWTER, LYMAN R. (1935). EQUINE ENCEPHALOMYELITIS CROSS-IMMUNITY IN HORSES BETWEEN WESTERN AND EASTERN STRAINS OF VIRUS. SUPPLEMENTAL REPORT. Amer. Vet. Med. Assoc. Jour. 86 (n.s. 39): 773-777.

(49) ________VAWTER, LYMAN, and Others (1933). EQUINE ENCEPHALOMYELITIS. Nev. Agr. Expt. Sta. Bul. 132, 22 pp., illus.

(50) SCHOENING, H.W. (1939). EQUINE ENCEPHALOMYELITIS. Amer. Vet. Med. Assoc. Jour. 95: 268-271.

(51) ________(1940). THE EPIZOOTIOLOGY OF INFECTIOUS EQUINE ENCEPHALOMYELITIS IN THE UNITED STATES. Vet. Bul. 34 (1): 13-19.

(52) ________(1940). REACTIONS FOLLOWING ADMINISTRATION OF EQUINE ENCEPHALOMYELITIS VACCINE. Amer. Vet. Med. Assoc. Jour. 97: 39-40, illus.

(53) ________GILTNER, L.T., and SHAHAN, M.S. (1939). INFECTIOUS EQUINE ENCEPHALOMYELITIS IN 1939. U.S. Live Stock Sanit. Assoc. Proc. 43: 145-150.

(54) SOHOENING, H. W., SHAHAN, M.S., OSTEEN, O.L., and GILTNER, L.T. (19400. STUDIES ON THE INTRADERMAL METHOD OF VACCINATION AGAINST EQUINE ENCEPHALOMYELITIS. Vet. Med. 35: 377-380, illus.

(55) SCHWARTE, L.H., BIEBTER, H.E., and MURRAY, CHAS (1937). A DISEASE OF HORSES CAUSED BY FEEDING MOLDY CORN. Amer. Vet. Med. Assoc. Jour. 90 (n.s. 43): 76-85, illus.

(56) SHAHAN, M.S., and GILTNER, L.T. (1934). SOME ASPECTS OF INFECTION AND IMMUNITY IN EQUINE ENCEPHALOMYELITIS. Amer. Vet. Med. Assoc. Jour. 84 (n.s. 37): 928-934.

(57) ________and GILTNER, L.T. (1935). EQUINE ENCEPHALOMYELITIS STUDIES: 1. CROSS-IMMUNITY TESTS BETWEEN EASTERN AND WESTERN TYPES OF VIRUS. Amer. Vet. Med. Assoc. Jour. 86 (n.s. 39): 764-772.

(58) ________GILTNER, L.T., DAVIS, C.L. and HUFFMAN, W.T. (1939). "SEONDARY DISEASE" OCCURRING SUBSEQUENT TO INFECTIOUS EQUINE ENCEPHALOMYELITIS. Vet. Med. 34: 354-358, illus.

(59) ________GILTNER, L.T., and OSTEEN, C.L. (1940). THE ISOLATION AND TYPING OF EQUINE ENCEPHALOMYELITIS VIRUS. Cornell Vet. 30: 151-160.

(60) ________GILTNER, L.T., and SCHOENING, H.W. (1938). A REVIEW OF THE 1938 OUTBREAK OF INFECTIOUS EQUINE ENCEPHALOMYELITIS IN THE UNITED STATES. U.S. Live Stock Sanit. Assoc. Proc.42: 45-157.

(61) SIMMONS, JAMES STEVENS, REYNOLDS, FRANCOIs H.K., and CORNELL, VIRGIL H. (19360. TRANSMISSION OF THE VIRUS OF EQUINE ENCEPHALOMYELITIS THROUGH AEDES ALBOPICTUS, SKUZE. Amer. Jour. Trop. Med. 16: 289-302.

(62) SYVERTON, JEROME T. (1940). DISCUSSION ON EPIDEMIOLOGY OF EQUINE ENCEPHALOMYELITIS. Internatl. Cong. Microbiol. Proc. 3: 306.

(63) ________and BERRY, GEORGE PACKER (1936). AN ARTHROPOD VECTOR FOR EQUINE ENCEPHALOMYELITIS, WESTERN STRAIN. Science 84: 186-187.

(64) ________and BERRY, GEORGE PACKER (1941). HEREDITARY TRANSMISSION OF THE WESTERN TYPE OF EQUINE ENCEPHALOMYELITIS VIRUS IN THIS WOOD TICK, DERMACENTOR ANDERBONI STILES. Jour. Expt. Med. 73: 507-530, illus.

(65) TEN BROECK, CARL (1938). BIRDS AS POSSIBLE CABRIEBS OF THE VIRUS OF EQUINE ENCEPHALOMYELITIS. Arch. Path. 25: 759.

(66) ________HURST, E. WESTON, and TRAUB, EBICH (1935). EPIDEMIOLOGY OF EQUINE ENCEPHALOMYELITIS IN THE EASTERN UNITED STATES. Jour. Expt. Med. 62: 677-685, illus.

(67) ________and MERRTT. T., MALOOLY H. (1933). A SEROLOGICAL DIFFERENCE BETWEEN EASTERN AND WESTERN EQUINE ENCEPHALOMYELITIS VIRUS. Soc. Expt. Biol. and Med. Proc. 31: 217-220.

(68) UNITED STATES BUREAU OF ANIMAL INDUSTRY (1933). RESEARCH ON DISEASES. In Rpt. of the Chief of the Bur. of Anim. Indus. 1933: 33-34.

(69) ________(1934). RESEARCH ON DISEASES. In Rpt. of the Chief of the Bur. of Anim. Indus. 1934: 37-38.

(70) ________(1938). INFECTIOUS EQUINE ENCEPHALOMYELITIS AND BELATED DISEASES. In Rpt. of the Chief of the Bur. Anim. Indus. 1938: 58-59.

(71) ________(1941). REPORT OF THE CHIEF OF THE BUREAU OF ANIMAL INDUSTRY 92 pp.

(72) WEBSTER, LESLIE T., and WRIGHT, F. HOWELL (1938). RECOVERY OF EASTERN EQUINE ENCEPHALOMYELITIS VIRUS IN BRAIN TISSUE OF HUMAN CASES OF ENCEPHALITIS IN MASSACHUSETTS. Science 88: 305-306.

Chapter 2

EQUINE INFECTIOUS ANEMIA OR SWAMP FEVER

C.D. Stein[1]

[1] *C.D. Stein is Veterinarian, Pathological Division, Bureau of Animal Industry*

Human beings have their malaria and horses their swamp fever, but the latter is the mote difficult to diagnose and treat. The horse disease is widespread, persistent, and debilitating, and the virus has been known to remain active in an animal for many years. The author suggests practical ways to minimize the damage.

Infectious anemia or swamp fever, also known in some sections of the United States as malarial fever, slow fever, and mountain fever, is one of the most serious maladies of the horse, and because of its insidious nature and widespread distribution it has become a problem of world-wide concern.

Infectious anemia is an acute or chronic disease of equines, caused by a filtrable virus that poisons the blood and characterized principally by intermittent fever, marked depression, progressive weakness, loss of weight, edema (dropsy like swelling), congestion and icterus (jaundice) of the visible mucous membranes, and anemia of a transitory or progressive type.

Long recognized as a specific infectious disease of equines, infectious anemia was reported from Europe as early as 1843. It occurs in various parts of Europe, Asia, Africa, and North America (*9*).[2] Recently the disease has been reported from Venezuela, South America. The disease has existed in the United States for at least 50 years, and since 1900 has been authentically reported in isolated areas from 29 States. In 15 of these States the virus was recovered by horse-inoculation tests, while diagnosis in the other 14 States was based oil clinical examination. Since 1932, outbreaks of the disease have been reported from Maryland, Massachusetts, Mississippi, New York, Indiana, Illinois, Michigan, Kansas, Wyoming, Montana, Colorado, Oregon, Idaho, Texas, Virginia, Vermont, and Washington. Since 1935 investigators in the Bureau of Animal Industry have isolated the virus from field cases in New York, Maryland, Virginia, Mississippi, Louisiana, Pennsylvania, California, Texas, and Wyoming.

Because of the difficulty of diagnosis, the disease is probably more widespread than the reports indicate. Generally speaking, it is most prevalent in poorly drained, low-lying sections, but it has been found in wooded sections and on marshy pastures at high altitudes. It also appears to be more prevalent when biting insects are most numerous and during wet years. The disease appears in the active form in May or June and reaches its height in midsummer, usually declining late in the fall. Chronic cases may be seen at all seasons of the year, and it is possible to produce the disease experimentally at any time.

Except in the Mississippi Delta, the disease occurs in the United States mostly as a sporadic infection, isolated cases or outbreaks for the most part being reported from and confined to low-lying and wooded sections in the States where it is known to exist. In the Mississippi Delta the disease has become established among the mules on the large cotton plantations and is of considerable economic importance; occurring principally in the chronic form, it saps the strength of the animals and renders them incapable of regular work in the busy cotton-growing season when they are most needed (*5*).

Cause

Studies and observations of the disease made by Bureau of Animal Industry investigators in the field and under experimental

---

[2] Italic numbers in parentheses refer to Literature Cited.

conditions indicate that debilitating influences that lower the resistance of an animal, such as overexertion, extreme heat, high humidity, faulty nutrition; improper care and handling, bad sanitation, impure water supply, and a heavy infestation of intestinal parasites, are not only predisposing factors but also have a marked influence on the progress of the disease in infected animals. Gates (5) in 1939, reporting on the disease in Mississippi, made similar observations.

Although the infectious nature of the disease was known as early as 1859, the causative agent was not definitely established until 1904, when Carre and Vallee (2) demonstrated that it was a filtrable virus. This finding was confirmed by the early investigations of the Bureau and has since been repeatedly substantiated.

Under natural conditions the virus appears to be specific for equines (the horse, mule, and donkey). It may persist in the host for years. It is apparently present in the blood and body tissues of affected animals at all times and may be eliminated with some of the secretions or excretions. The disease can be readily transmitted experimentally to equines by inoculation, beneath the skin or into the blood stream, of whole blood, blood serum, or spleen, brain or other tissue emulsions. Experiments and transmission tests made by the Bureau with strains of virus isolated from widely separated areas indicate that its virulence is exceedingly variable and appears to be influenced by a number of factors. Among these are the individual susceptibility of the host, frequency of passage–that is, transmission of the disease from one animal to another (in series) at short intervals–method of exposure, source of virus, character of the inoculating substance (inoculum), and debilitating factors affecting the host.

The virus shows considerable resistance against disinfectants, heating, freezing, and drying. Definite findings of Bureau investigators concerning the action of heat and chemicals on the virus have been put into practical use in formulating requirements for the treatment of antiserums prepared from horses, thus safeguarding against dissemination of swamp fever through the use of such biological products. Biological supply houses operating under Government license are now required to heat all antiserums prepared from horses at 58° to 59°C. (136.4° to 138.2°F.) for an hour, which destroys any infectious anemia virus they may contain.

Dissemination and Transmission

While dissemination of the disease usually follows the introduction of infected animals into noninfected territory, the common method of transmission in the natural state is not definitely known. Ordinarily the disease appears to spread slowly. During the transportation of great numbers of horses, however, outbreaks may occur when infected animals are moved into new territory where conditions are favorable for transmission and for the exposure of large numbers of normal horses.

A number of investigators who have worked on this problem are of the opinion that the disease is spread principally in pastures where the virus-laden urine and feces of infected animals contaminate the feed and water, but the part that biting insects may play under these conditions cannot be ignored.,

Experimental evidence indicates:

(1) That the disease is readily transmitted by the injection of blood or tissue emulsions from affected animals into susceptible ones;

(2) That minute doses of the virus are infective for susceptible animals;

(3) That the body secretions or excretions may contain the virus;

(4) That infected mares may transmit the disease to their offspring;

(5) That the disease may be transmitted by external parasites, including biting flies and biting lice;

(6) That it may spread slowly by long, continuous, intimate contact; and

(7) That carriers probably constitute one of the most common sources of the virus in nature and are chiefly concerned in the perpetuation of the disease. In adopting control measures, these factors should all be taken into consideration.

Infectious anemia has been reported in man in a few instances, but it is probable that man is not very susceptible to the disease. Verge (*10*) In 1933 reported the occurrence of two cases in human beings, those of Luhrs in 1920 and Peters in 1924. In the experiments conducted by the Bureau, equines only were found to be susceptible. Attempts to infect calves, sheep, swine, dogs, rabbits, guinea pigs, rats, mice, and pigeons were without success. Similar results have been obtained by various workers (*4*). Some investigators in foreign countries, however, have reported that a few other species, including young goats, pigs, rabbits, rats, chickens, and doves, can be infected under experimental conditions.

Mules appear to be somewhat more resistant than horses, acquiring the disease mostly in the chronic form. Balozet (*1*), in 1933, reported from Tunis, North Africa, that the African ass was as susceptible to the virus of infectious anemia as the horse but that the symptoms were more apparent in the horse. DeKock (*3*) reported a natural outbreak of infectious anemia in donkeys in Natal, South Africa, that assumed a rather virulent character.

Forms of the Disease, Symptoms, and Termination

The clinical symptoms are variable and depend to a great extent on the form the disease assumes. Infectious anemia may occur as an acute, rapidly fatal disease or, more commonly, as a chronic affection characterized by intermittent attacks of fever, loss of weight, progressive weakness, marked depression, and dropsical swellings on the lower portions of the body and on the legs. The disease may also exist in a form in which no clinical symptoms are apparent though the affected animal carries virulent virus in the blood stream.

In the acute form of the disease the incubation period following subcutaneous injection (beneath the skin) of infected blood is usually about 12 to 15 days, though it may vary from less than a week to 3 months and possibly longer. The onset is sudden and is manifested by a rise in temperature, which usually goes to about 105° F, but may reach 108°. In the acute form the febrile attacks are usually severe and may be more or less continuous or very frequent. In this connection it should be mentioned that the irregular recurrent fever is one of the chief clinical manifestations of the disease, and in mild cases it sometimes constitutes the only symptom. Respiration is accelerated and frequently is of the abdominal type. The animal is dejected, the head hangs low, leg weakness is marked, the body weight is shifted from one leg to another, and the hind feet are frequently placed well forward under the body. The membranes of the eyès s1iow congestion, followed by brownish to yellowish discoloration. Feed is refused. There may be a slight watery discharge from the eyes and nose and, if the weather is extremely warm, profuse sweating. Frequent urination may also be noted and in severe cases diarrhoea may develop. The attack usually lasts from 3 to 5 days, after which the temperature returns to normal and the animal appears to be well except for a marked loss of weight. Occasionally, however, the initial attack may persist until the animal dies.

Dropsical swellings of the sheath, the legs, the chest, and the under surfaces of the body may occur at any time. These frequently disappear and appear again at the same or other places. Subsequent attacks usually follow, with intervening periods of normality varying from a few days to many weeks or months. When the intervals between the attacks of fever are short, the animal seldom lives more than 15 to 30 days. During the attacks of fever and immediately afterward, there is a reduction in the number of red corpuscles in the blood. When this is pronounced, it can be readily demonstrated by drawing some blood into a test tube in the bottom of which a small amount of powdered potassium oxalate or other anticoagulant has been placed to prevent clotting. During the bleeding process the tube should be agitated gently to mix the blood with the anticoagulant. The tube containing the blood sample should be placed in an upright position to permit the red corpuscles to gravitate to the bottom, and after half an hour a comparison of the sedimented red corpuscles with a sample similarly drawn from a normal horse will clearly demonstrate the degree of anemia that exists. During the periods of normality between attacks, the red-corpuscle count is in a great majority of cases normal.

The subacute and chronic forms of the disease differ from the acute in that the attacks are less severe and the intervals between them are longer. The subacute cases may terminate in death during following one of the attacks, or the reactions may grow less frequent, the animal finally developing into a chronic case or a clinically recovered carrier. In general, the chronic form is manifested by unthriftiness, rough coat, underweight, sluggishness, weakness, dropsical swelling of the lower parts of the body or on the legs; muddy discoloration of the visible mucous membranes, and small hemorrhages on the nictitating membrane (the third eyelid, or haw) and the nasal septum (the partition between the passages of the nose).

As the disease progresses, evidence of anemia may develop, the red-corpuscle count may be extremely low, the blood may appear thin and watery, and in the later stages the visible mucous membranes may become pallid. The pulse may be slow and weak, the heart action may become irregular, and a jugular pulse may be visible. There may be a rapid slowing of the pulse after exercise. Muscular weakness is manifested by a wobbly or rolling staggering gait or by partial paralysis of the hindquarters. In the chronic form of the disease the appetite is for the most part unimpaired and frequently is ravenous, so that the animals may eat continuously if they have access to feed. In spite of the excessive consumption of feed, however, there is a progressive loss of body weight (Fig. 1).

Animals affected with this form of the disease can perform some work if handled with care. They are subject, however, to recurring attacks characterized by extreme weakness, knuckling, inability to walk in a straight line, and prominent hemorrhages on the third eyelid. The weakness may become so great that the animal cannot

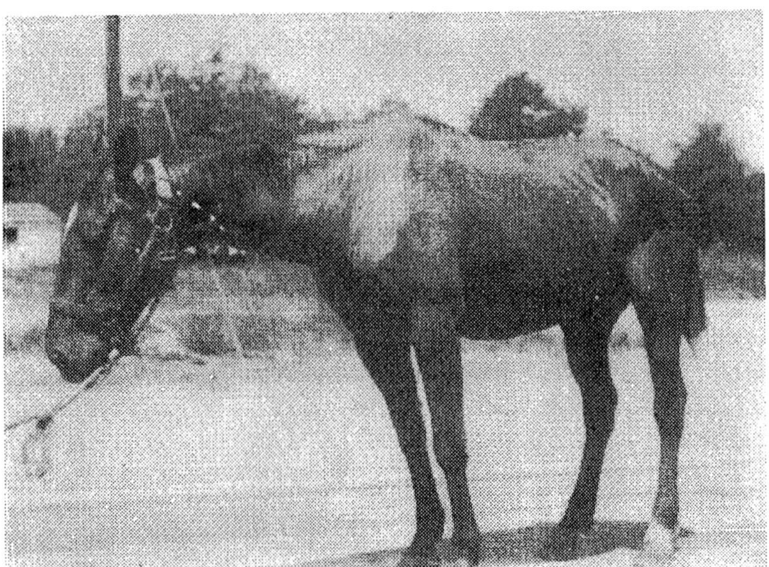

Fig. 1: The poor condition of this horse is the result of infectious anaemia in the chronic form.

stand without support. With good attention, rest, and supportive treatment, it usually overcomes these periodic attacks and may go back to routine work. Each attack takes its toll of flesh and strength, however, and repetitions, if frequent enough, will so weaken the animal as to render it useless or finally bring about death by exhaustion.

The inactive or latent form of the disease may follow the initial attack, but it is usually preceded by several attacks of fever. This form is observed in animals that have apparently recovered from the acute, subacute, or chronic types of the disease. Animals affected with the disease in the latent form show no clinical symptoms and are known as clinically recovered carriers. The temperature remains normal, and there is no reduction in the red corpuscles or any sign of disease over a period of years, and yet the infectious agent is always present in the blood stream and all the tissues and may be eliminated with the body excretions. Such animals obviously are a menace to other horses that may be near them, since they are veritable reservoirs of infection that for the most part go unrecognized and uncontrolled. The inactive form of the disease may, however, become active at any time and present all the characteristics of the acute or subacute form. Unusually hard work or any debilitating influence may reactivate the infection.

The Bureau of Animal Industry has under observation a horse that is a good example of the inactive form of infectious anemia. This horse was exposed to the disease August 2, 1935, by being given, an injection of filtered blood from two horses known to have infectious anemia. After an incubation period of 12 days, a typical attack of fever occurred, which in turn was followed by two more attacks within a 3-week period. No further attacks occurred over a period of approximately 5 years. During this time the animal remained in good physical condition and showed no symptoms of disease whatever; yet blood drawn from it at intervals during the 5 years produced infectious anemia when injected into normal horses. A horse with a similar history that has been infected for approximately 6 years is also being held under observation; although this animal has shown no clinical symptoms for more than 6 years its blood remains infectious.

Schalk and Roderick (7), of the North Dakota Agricultural Experiment Station, and Scott (*8*), of the Wyoming station, have reported inactive cases that were infectious over even longer periods.

Heath (*6*) in 1931, reporting on transmission experiments carried on apparently during 1930, presented evidence to show that blood from an immune carrier (a mare originally infected in 1912), when injected intravenously into normal horses, produced infectious anemia in the subacute form.

Anatomical Changes

The pathological alterations in the body tissues resulting from artificially induced infectious anemia are extremely variable. The changes may be very well marked and plainly visible (in some cases so pronounced as to be striking), or they may be so slight as to escape detection except by those having considerable experience with the disease. The lesions, which may occur in any degree of intensity or in any combination, are most commonly observed in acute and subacute cases and in chronic cases dying during an acute flare-up.

The most constant lesions of swamp fever are hemorrhages of varying sizes on the serous and mucous membranes of the body, with enlargement and other changes of the spleen, kidneys, liver, and heart. The hemorrhages are most frequently found on the parietal and visceral pleura, the pericardium, epicardium, and endocardium, the parietal and visceral peritoneum, the mucosa of the small and large intestines, the mucosa of the caecum, and the surface of the spleen and kidneys.

The spleen for the most part is enlarged. Occasionally it will be found to be approximately three times its normal size, and the splenic pulp will be soft and blackish red in color. The liver is frequently enlarged to enormous proportions and is hard and friable. It may vary from a yellowish-brown, cooked appearance to a reddish brown. Frequently there is pigmentation of a yellowish-brown or greenish-gray tinge. In cross section the lobules stand out quite prominently, presenting a nutmeglike appearance. The kidneys are frequently enlarged, edematous, and lighter in color than normal, and they show numerous hemorrhages on the surface ranging from the size of a pin point to several millimeters in diameter. The heart may be enlarged, flabby, and lighter in color than normal, or it may have a cooked appearance, and it shows hemorrhages over the epicardium, in the myocardium, and on the endocardium. The heart fat frequently loses its normal consistency and color and becomes soft and gelatinous. The visceral lymph glands are usually enlarged and edematous and may be impregnated with hemorrhages. Large areas of hemorrhages are found in the marrow of the long bones, especially of the femur. Yellowish discoloration of the connective tissues and fat may also be evident. As stated before, the lesions are quite variable.

In those subacute or chronic cases showing clinical manifestations of a progressive anemia, the autopsy may also show pale mucous membranes and light-colored, thin, watery blood.

For the most part the tissue changes found in the acute and subacute cases are more extensive and more pronounced than those in the chronic cases. In chronic cases terminating in death from exhaustion following a protracted illness, lesions indicative of cachexia (general ill health) are usually observed, such as emaciation, gelatinous infiltration of connective tissue and fat tissue, especially the fat tissue of the heart, and a blanched appearance of mucous membranes. In such cases the hemorrhagic infiltration of tissues and degenerative changes of the organs may be very slight or entirely absent.

In latent cases (symptomless carriers) and chronic cases of a mild type little or no anatomical alteration is observed on autopsy. The most constant and characteristic histopathological findings are round-cell infiltration and a heavy deposition of hemosiderin in the liver and spleen. The post mortem histological findings are of considerable assistance in making a tentative diagnosis.

Diagnosis

Diagnosis of infectious anemia is usually a difficult matter, since there are no symptoms or post mortem changes that can be considered characteristic or peculiar to this disease alone. The only definite means of diagnosis is by horse-inoculation test. Considering collectively the history of the case, clinical symptoms, and blood examinations, diagnosis with a reasonable degree of accuracy can possibly be made in the active form of the disease. For example, a history of rapid loss of flesh, loss of spirit and energy, evidences of muscular weakness with intermittent attacks of fever, congestion of the mucous membranes of the eye, with possibly some degree of jaundice, and dropsical swellings of the lower parts of the body, collectively, are strongly suggestive of infectious anemia. The tentative diagnosis will be further strengthened if during and immediately after the febrile period an examination of the blood shows a diminution in the volume of the red corpuscles, an increase in the rate at which they gravitate, and a decrease of hemoglobin. It must be remembered, however, that in the intervals between the attacks of fever the blood picture, except in cases accompanied by a progressive anemia, usually returns to normal.

Infectious anemia in the inactive form would ordinarily not be detected, since no clinical symptoms would be present to cause suspicion. It should be remembered also that heavy infestation with intestinal parasites, especially strongyles, produces symptoms that are in some respects similar to those of infectious anemia. Microscopic examinations of the feces for the eggs of these parasites and examination of blood films for evidence of eosinophilia (an increase in the number of certain white blood corpuscles) will assist in making a differential diagnosis. It is possible, and in some areas probable, that some horses and mules will be heavily infested with intestinal parasites and at the same time have chronic infectious anemia.

In acute cases occurring in the field, death may occur before the usual train of symptoms develops. The disease in the acute form may be confused with anthrax, influenza, purpura hemorrhagica, acute equine encephalomyelitis, and other acute febrile conditions. In the subacute and chronic forms it may be mistaken for trypanosomiasis (dourine, murrina, and surra) or strongylidosis.

Since the development of practical and reliable means of diagnosis is of primary importance from the standpoint of control, a considerable amount of experimental work on diagnostic procedures has been carried out by the Bureau of Animal Industry. No laboratory blood test was found sufficiently satisfactory to warrant its adoption as a standard diagnostic method, and antigens prepared from the blood, tissues, and urine of affected animals failed to produce a specific response of diagnostic value.

Treatment and Control

Many investigators have unsuccessfully tried to treat the disease with various agents such as arsenic preparations, quinine, various dyes, mercurial preparations, and a number of others. In sections where the disease is endemic, or constantly present, practicing veterinarians employ supportive treatment, using arsenical compounds; principally sodium cacodylate, together with tonics, rest, and abundance of good feed, at the same time eliminating intestinal parasites and other, debilitating factors. While such treatment brings about some clinical improvement, it has no lasting value, for the animal remains infected, is subject to febrile attacks, and is a virus carrier. To establish a complete cure, a method of treatment must be found that will not only free the animal of clinical symptoms but completely eliminate the virus from the tissues.

The control of this disease, because of its obscure nature, the difficulty of diagnosis, its resistance to treatment, and its widespread distribution, presents a problem of serious concern to all owners of horses and mules, especially those with a large number of animals.

Preventive vaccination has been attempted without success by a number of investigators, including those in the Bureau of Animal Industry.

The control of infectious anemia depends primarily on the identification of the chronic carriers. While no systematic programme can be undertaken until a definite and practical means of diagnosis of chronic carriers is developed, the results of studies by Bureau and other investigators indicate that the following measures constitute the most effective means of control.

When a definite diagnosis of infectious anemia has been made, it is advisable, if practicable, to kill the animal and dispose of the carcass by cremation or deep burial to prevent further spread of the infection. This method of control has been followed in small isolated outbreaks and in establishments keeping large numbers of horses, and it has been effective in preventing the spread of the disease. It is obvious, however, that the method is impracticable in such areas as the Mississippi Delta, where the disease is widely distributed and exists principally in a mild chronic form.

Animals known to be infected and those suspected of having the disease should be isolated from healthy animals.

The common use of equipment that may produce skin abrasions or absorb body excretions or secretions, such its bridles, harness, saddles, blankets, brushes, and currycombs, on both infected and healthy horses is dangerous and should be avoided.

The greatest care should always be used to prevent transmission of the disease from animal to animal by the use of unsterilized instruments, bleeding needles, or hypodermic needles.

Since infected mares may transmit the disease to their offspring, such animals should not be used for breeding purposes.

Infected and healthy animals should not be kept together in small, poorly drained paddocks adjacent to stables and manure dumps.

Where premises are badly contaminated, or a number of cases of the disease have developed on certain pastures, it is advisable to move the animals to new quarters, deeply plow the ground, and fence off the infected areas. Horses or mules should not be permitted on such pastures or premises for at least 6 months.

The maintenance of good sanitary conditions, fly control, systematic control of intestinal parasites, and provision for a supply of pure, fresh drinking water should also receive attention, and under no circumstances should animals be permitted to drink from stagnant pools.

Literature Cited

(1) BALOZET, L. (1935). SENSIBILITE DE L'ANE AFRICAN A L'INOCULATION DU VIRUS DE L'ANEMIE INFECTIEUSE. Soc. de Biol. [Paris] Compt. Rend. 119: 62-65.

(2) CARRE, [H. J.], and VALLEE, [H. P.] (1904). SUR L'ANEMIE INFECTIEUSE DU CHEV Ah Acad. des Sci. [Paris] Compt. Rend. 139: 1239-1241.

(3) DEKOCK, G.V.D.W. (1924). A CONTRIBUTION TO THE STUDY OF THE VIRUS, HAEMATOLOGY AND PATHOLOGY OF INFECTIOUS ANAEMIA OF EQUINES UNDER SOUTH AFRICAN CONDITIONS. Union of So. Africa Dept. Agr. Rpts. 9 and 10 of the Dir. of Vet. Ed. and Res., 1923, pp. [253]-313, illus.

(4) FRANCIS, M., and MARSTELLER, R.P. (1908). INFECTIOUS ANEMIA OF THE HORSE. Tex. Agr. Expt. Sta. Bul. 119, 19 pp., illus.

(5) GATES, WILLIAM L. (1940). EQUINE INFECTIOUS ANEMIA (SWAMP FEVER). Amer. Vet. Med. Assoc. Jour. 96: 195-199.

(6) HEATH, L.M. (1931). RESEARCH ON SWAMP FEVER OR INFECTIOUS EQUINE ANAEMIA. Canada Dept. Agr. Rpt. Vet. Dir. Gen. (1931), App. 4, Path. Div. Rpt., pp. 70-71.

(7) SCHALK, A.F., and RODERICK, L.M. (1923). HISTORY OF A "SWAMP FEVER" VIRUS CARRIER. N. Dak. Agr. Expt. Sta. Bul. 168, 14 pp., illus.

(8) SCOTT, J.W. (1931). SWAMP FEVER IN HORSES. Wyo. Agr. Expt. Sta. Ann. Rpt. (1930-31) 41: 38.

(9) TORRANCE, F. (1902). REPORT ON "SWAMP FEVER" IN HORSES. Canada Min. of Agr. Ann. Rpt. 1901-2, p. 135.

(10) VERGE, J. (1933). L'ANEMIE INFECTIEUSE DES EQUIDES, MALADIE DE VALLEE. Rec. de Med. vet. 109: [797]-838, iilus.

Chapter 3

PERIODIC OPHTHALMIA OF HORSES

L.O. Mott & H.R. Seibold[1]

[1] *L.O. Mott and H.R. Seibold are Assistant Veterinarians, Pathological Division, Bureau of Animal Industry.*

Some experts estimate that 1 out of every 10, horses and mules in the United States is affected with moon blindness–a recurrent inflammation of the eyes that may end in loss of sight. It has been known for over 2,000 years, but no one yet knows the cause, or how to prevent or cure it. Here is the most recent scientific information about the disease and advice on treatment.

Periodic Ophthalmia, or moon blindness is a disease of the eye affecting horses, mules, and asses only. Its history dates back more than 2,000 years. The disease was studied in the earliest days of veterinary medicine. Vegetius wrote about it in the fourth century. During the early parts of the eighteenth century several famous veterinarians described the disease and recorded interesting facts about it. Research on a scientific basis, started as early as the latter part of the same century, has been continued up to the present time.

Distribution

Available literature records the presence of periodic ophthalmia in England, Germany, France, Italy, South Africa, the Philippine Islands, Central America, and North America. The geographical distribution is probably much more widespread, however; than the literature indicates, because the disease does not cause the death of animals and therefore in most countries is not listed as one of the reportable diseases. Difficulty in diagnosing the disease, together with lack of more complete knowledge regarding its cause, prevention, and treatment has given horse owners a somewhat hopeless outlook regarding it. While it continues to exist, it is seldom reported, and its true economic importance is unknown and probably underestimated.

In England it is reported that previous to 1880 the disease was very prevalent but that it has almost disappeared following the establishment of the Royal Commission on the Horse Breeding Industry, which brought about the condemnation for breeding purposes of all sires exhibited at shows if they had the slightest eye abnormality or any other ailment. This is achieved by rigid veterinary inspection.

Germany, France, and Italy have had the disease in a severe epizootic form. In those countries it appeared to be very closely associated with a low altitude. This point was especially noted in the German army during the transferring of horses. The number of horses with diseased eyes decreased or increased according to the altitude of the locality where the horses were stationed. Early cases often remained stationary or apparently recovered following the move to an unaffected area.

In France also the absence of the condition in areas of high altitude was noted, and some extensive experiments with normal young colts were carried out. Some animals from the high altitude were moved to different low altitudes, and animals from low altitudes were moved to high altitudes, with groups of native colts at each altitude retained as control animals. About 50 percent of the animals in the low altitudes became affected, both in the retained and the moved groups, whereas the disease did not appear in the groups at the high altitudes.

During the Boer War, Great Britain purchased a large number of horses and mules from the United States and transported them to South Africa. Within 2 years following the war, 14 percent of these animals had developed periodic ophthalmia. In certain remount stations the incidence of the disease was as high as 48 percent; at the same time a lower percentage of the native animals were affected.

The condition had not previously existed in South Africa. Later it gradually disappeared., so that now this region is free of the disease and has been for 30 years.

Panama, which is now reported to have about the same amount of the disease as the United States, until the last 8 years was relatively free of it. It does not exist in Hawaii, but in the Philippine Islands it appears to be almost tour times as prevalent as in continental United States.

The disease has been reported to be of little economic importance in Canada.

The disease seems to occur seldom in the western part of the United States: From reports of various surveys made, a line drawn through the middle of the Dakotas, Nebraska, Kansas, Oklahoma, and Texas would about determine its western limit. Almost all of the States east of this line have the disease, and it affects animals at both high and low altitudes.

Prevallence

It is rather difficult to estimate the incidence of the disease or the annual economic loss it causes in the United States, but both are undoubtedly very large. Some investigators have estimated that as many as 10 percent of the horses and mules in this country are affected. Limited field investigations conducted by the Bureau of Animal Industry indicate that the incidence of the disease in some of the Middle Atlantic States is much higher than was generally supposed. The rate of incidence in different areas covered varied from 0 to as high as 30 percent. The variation on farms in different areas appears to be closely correlated with the concentration of animals, a higher percentage of affected animals being found on highly productive soils and good farms where more horses and mules are used than on the scattered farms with poor soil, where the percentage of affected animals almost always dropped very noticeably.

A very conservative estimate would set the monetary loss at least at half a million dollars annually.

Theories about the Cause

The cause of periodic ophthalmia is unknown, but theories about it are numerous. Among other superstitions is the idea that wolf teeth are responsible, and to this day many wolf teeth are extracted to satisfy owners who still hold to this idea. Many horsemen discriminate against the use of blind stallions on the ground that the condition itself, or more likely a weakness or predisposition to the disease, is inherited. One investigator cites a stallion 90 to 95 percent of whose offspring contracted the disease, most of them becoming affected at between 3 and 8 years of age. Other investigators have reported that the condition affects one generation and then misses one or more generations before appearing again. Data accumulated by the Bureau of Animal Industry on a recent field survey indicate the possibility of hereditary susceptibility to the disease.

The association of the disease with low altitudes in foreign countries and its absence in the western part of the United States suggest some correlation with environment. However, comparison of accumulated data from farms free of the disease with similar data from farms where it developed, all within an affected area covered by the Bureau of Animal Industry's survey, showed no correlation with environment. This is slight evidence, however, because the farms free of the disease and those on which It existed were both in the same area.

The possibility that nutritional deficiencies, glandular disturbances, or parasites are directly or indirectly responsible for the disease cannot be overlooked in future investigations.

The infection theory has been investigated by many noted scientists who have worked on the disease. Several research workers have introduced a disease that resembled periodic ophthalmia by inoculations within the eye, but they failed to secure a recurrence of attacks. In one instance the disease was reported to have been transmitted from animal to animal by the use of germ-free filtrates made from the eyes of active cases. Such findings would point to a filterable virus as the causative factor, but the work has not been confirmed.

As observed in field investigations carried on by the Bureau of Animal Industry, the disease has all the appearances of an infectious one. It usually appears sporadically within a community or area, sometimes affecting only a few farms and sometimes farms in several counties, but most often affecting from 5 to 30 percent of the animals, within a year or two of the same date. Very often following this sporadic appearance of the disease, it will subside and no new cases, will develop for years even when blind animals continue to live on the farms., If the condition again occurs, it almost always does so sporadically. On some farms the disease appears to be more persistent, affecting new animals year after year. These cases are relatively uncommon, but they make the picture still more confused.

The fact that the attacks are accompanied by mild fever, localized severe inflammation followed by abatement of acute symptoms, atrophy, and degeneration of the eyeball, together with the field observations mentioned, makes the infection theory seem plausible.

Lesions and Anatomical Changed

Clinically, the condition is primarily a disease of the eyes. Various authors have suggested the presence of other clinical symptoms and post mortem findings associated with it, but these have not as yet been generally accepted. It is characterized by a recurring inflammation which may affect one eye alone, or both eyes either simultaneously or alternately, or one eye until blindness occurs and then the other eye. The onset of the attack is sudden, usually being noticed first in the morning, the animal having appeared normal the night before. The eyelids are swollen and tender, and the eye is kept closed. A watery discharge runs from the eyes. There is some rise of body temperature, accompanied by other evidences of a generalized disturbance. After a week or 10 days the inflammation subsides, and the eye or eyes either may appear to be little affected or may be chalk white and completely blind. The Interval between attacks may vary from a few weeks to several months, and the number of attacks may vary from 1 to 10 or 20, occurring over a period of years.

Blindness following early attacks is usually due to adhesions of the iris to the lens. If these adhesions break down before they are attached too firmly, the lens will usually clear. Following the earlier attacks, an examination of the eye with an ophthalmoscope (an instrument for viewing the interior of the eye) will reveal only a partial opacity or opaque spots on the lens and sometimes a totally cleared lens with practically normal vision.

The cornea or outside surface of the eye is usually cloudy (blue white) during an attack but almost always clears in a few days and usually remains clear even after the animal is totally blind, the chalk-white appearance of the blind eye being due to an opacity of the lens.

The fluid within the eye also presents a cloudy appearance during an attack. Following an attack, this fluid will sometimes slowly clear, often presenting a hazy appearance for weeks following. Frequently an agglutination or clumping of cells within the eye fluid takes place, which looks like sediment or strings floating around, whenever disturbed by movement of the head.

The optic disk and retina are less often available for examination in most affected eyes because of other opaque structures in front of, them, but in cases where vision is clear or partly clear very little if any change is noticeable.

Diagnosis

The diagnosis of periodic ophthalmia is very difficult, since the cause of the condition is unknown and no laboratory test or testing agent has been made available for diagnostic purposes. Ophthalmoscopic examination for the presence of cataracts, spots on the lens, and any other opacity or cloudiness is the best available method for recognizing an affected animal when little is known about the animal's source or past history. Where the animal's history is complete, a positive diagnosis is much more easily arrived at because of the characteristic attacks and the sporadic appearance of the condition in other animals within the community or the same stable.

A technical description of microscopic changes due to the disease is given at the end of this article. This is based on recent work in the Bureau of Animal Industry.

Susceptibility

There is little variation in the degree of susceptibility of animals of different types, breeds, or sex. Mules are reported to be less susceptible than horses, and the condition has been observed in asses. There is, however, a noticeable age factor. Most horses are 3 or 4 years old or older before they become affected, and the disease not uncommonly develops in horses between 15 and 20 years of age. A few cases develop in 2-year-olds, fewer in yearlings. Very few cases are recorded in sucklings between 6 months and 1 year old, and so far as is known there are no authentic cases recorded in newborn foals or those under 6 months of age.

It has been observed that no young animals under 3 years of age have ever been affected except where the disease, made its appearance in a severe epizootic form, affecting several older animals before the young became affected.

Prevention and Control

No preventive or curative measures have been discovered. Prompt attention to the attacks as they occur by a competent veterinarian may materially prolong the sight in the affected eye or eyes. Treatment consists of application of cold compresses to the eye; administration of drugs to dilate the pupil, followed by drugs to contract the pupil, in order to prevent adhesions of the iris to the cornea or to the crystal-line lens; and mild laxatives to decrease the pressure within the eye-ball indirectly. The animal should be at complete rest in a partly darkened stable.

Intravenous injections of foreign proteins, such as sterile milk and typhoid vaccine, and other products, including some of the salts of arsenic, mercury, and iodine, when used in the early stages of the disease often shorten the period of an attack and help to prolong the sight.

Horsemen and breeders who hope to ward off this disease from their animals could practice no more sound control, considering the present lack of knowledge of its infectiousness and inheritance, than to keep their animals isolated from any possible direct or indirect contact with affected animals and discourage the breeding of affected animals.

Histopathology–Technical Description

Although numerous clinical and bacteriological investigations of periodic ophthalmia have been made in the past, histopathological (microscopic) study of this disease has been undertaken only recently. This has been due in part to the technical difficulties encountered in the microscopic examination of diseased equine eyes.

The microscopic lesions of periodic ophthalmia consist of inflammatory and degenerative changes that progress with the course of the disease. The early stages are characterized by iridocyclitis, or inflammation of the ciliary body and iris. The blood vessels of the ciliary body and iris become congested, and large numbers of lymphocytes and plasma cells are found in the connective tissue stroma of these structures. The nonpigmented ciliary epithelium that covers the ciliary processes exhibits marked changes. These epithelial cells become taller than normal. Brush like bundles of coarse fibrillar structures that stain red with eosin appear within the confines of this layer of cells. These fibrillar structures extend in a direction parallel with the nuclei of the cells and can best be demonstrated with differential staining techniques: Large numbers of lymphoid cells infiltrate between the individual cells of the non-pigmented ciliary epithelium. The general impression gained from these lesions is that the non-pigmented ciliary epithelium is the structure most seriously affected by the unknown agent of periodic ophthalmia at the onset of the disease.

In conjunction with the inflammatory lesions in the ciliary body and iris, the vitreous body and the aqueous humor exhibit changes in character. This is evidenced by the fact that both the aqueous humor and the vitreous body often coagulate after the eye has been placed in formalin instead of remaining watery in consistency. This change may be due to injury of the non-pigmented ciliary epithelium, which is thought to secrete a part of the fluid that occupies the spaces of the eyeball. Large numbers of lymphocytes and plasma cells are found in the vitreous body and aqueous humor and in the spaces between the fibers of the suspensory ligament of the lens (canals of Petit).

As a result of these inflammatory changes, the iris often becomes cemented to the lens (posterior synechia) or to the posterior surface of the cornea (anterior synechia), causing the "fixed pupil" so often encountered on clinical examination. This places the iris under considerable tension, frequently resulting in mechanical injury to the iris when the muscle fibers in this organ contract. Where anterior synechia has occurred, it is not uncommon to find evidence of mechanical injury at the posterior surface of the cornea, namely, rupture of Descemet's membrane and desquamation of the posterior endothelium.

As the disease progresses, the inflammation of the ciliary body becomes less acute. The coarse red fibrils in the non-pigmented ciliary epithelial layer become less numerous, but the cells do not return to their normal state. They may proliferate and assume an irregular arrangement. In some cases they swell to several times their normal size and assume a fine granular appearance. In many cases the ciliary body becomes covered with a fibrocellular inflammatory membrane. (cyclitie membrane).This membrane may envelop the posterior surface of the lens and extend across the entire diameter of the eye. A similar membrane may form anterior to the lens (pupillary membrane).

The lens becomes involved as the disease progresses. The lens fibers degenerate, and the epithelium of the lens proliferates, forming a complicated, capsulolenticular cataract. This type of cataract cannot be treated successfully by surgical methods. In many advanced cases the lens has undergone complete liquefaction, and only the capsule can be found on microscopic examination. The lens frequently becomes dislocated owing to injury to its suspensory ligament and to the non-pigmented ciliary epithelium to which this ligament is attached.

Changes in the retina occur simultaneously with changes in the lens. The retina may become completely or partially detached from the choroid coat, or it may remain in place. Regardless of its position, it degenerates. The rods cones (neuroepithelial elements), and ganglion cells disappear, but the supporting cells (glia cells) persist and may proliferate. Where the retina has become detached, it usually moves forward in the eye and comes to rest just behind. the lens. In these cases it may unite with the inflammatory membrane arising from the ciliary body and eventually form a wide band of fibrocellular tissue extending across the diameter of the eye.

As the retina degenerates, the optic nerve degenerates. In advanced chronic cases, nerve fibers cannot be demonstrated in the optic nerve. The funiculi of the nerve appear to be composed of masses of supporting neuroglia tissue (replacement gliosis). The optic nerve head and the nerve fiber layer of the retina are often infiltrated with lymphocytes and plasma cells.

The choroid coat may be congested and to some extent infiltrated with lymphocytes and plasma cells. In advanced cases the choroid appears thickened, perhaps as a result of shrinking of the eyeball.

Lesions of a minor character are found in the cornea. Small capillary blood vessels are often found in the proper substance of the cornea, particularly in the latter stages of the disease. The proper substance of the cornea usually contains an increased number of cellular elements just posterior to the corneal epithelium. The cellular elements consist of an increased number of corneal corpuscles, along with a varying number of polymorphonuclear leucocytes. In some advanced chronic cases the proper substance of the cornea appears thinner than normal.

Shrinking of the eyeball (phthisis bulbi) is a constant lesion of periodic ophthalmia. This is caused by a decreased tension of the ocular fluids, possibly a result of deranged function of the non pigmented ciliary epithelium. As the disease progresses, this shrinking and distortion of the eyeball is aggravated by contraction of the fibrocellular inflammatory membranes that so often form. In such cases the eyeball becomes greatly reduced in size, and the fundus may become completely filled with newly formed fibrocellular tissue.

Although the inflammatory lesions are most pronounced at the onset of the disease, the degenerative changes are of particular stgnificance. The latter appear to be most pronounced in the epithelial structures of the eye, namely, the non-pigmented epithelium of the ciliary body, the lens, and the neuroepithelial elements of the retina.

Chapter 4

GLANDERS

T.W. Cole[1]

[1] *T.W. Cole is Senior Veterinarian and Assistant Chief of the Field Inspection Division, Bureau of Animal Industry.*

During the war of 1914-18, the French Army lost enormous numbers of horses because of glanders. This is one of the serious diseases that has been practically eliminated in the United States. The job now is to see that it stays out of our country.

Glanders is a serious constitutional disease of equines (horses, asses, and mules) and occasionally of other animals and man. Formerly widespread in the United States, it has been virtually eradicated within the memory of the present generation. Fortunately most other farm animals, including cattle, sheep, goats, and swine, are for all practical purposes immune and require no special consideration in the control and eradication of this highly infectious malady. The disease is caused by a specific micro-organism called *Bacillus mallei* and is usually manifested by nodular lesions of the lungs and to a lesser degree of other organs, as well as by ulcerative lesions of the skin and the mucous membranes of the nasal cavity and respiratory passage. The term "farcy" is at times applied to the form of glanders in which the skin lesions are the more pronounced.

History

Few if any diseases have a more ancient recorded history. Glanders was recognized by Hippocrates about 450 B.C. and described with considerable accuracy by Apsyrtus, a Greek veterinarian of the time of Constantine the Great, who knew of its contagious character centuries before the microscope was invented. Down through history, war, with its concentration of horse stock, has been responsible for the greatest devastation by glanders. From time to time the Armies of Great Britain and the countries of continental Europe have suffered tremendous losses from the scourge. During the World War 1914-18, in the French Army alone over 58,000 animals were officially declared glanderous. Many of these were slaughtered and used for food, but the loss of work stock was enormous.

According to the best information available, the disease was imported into the United States at the close of the eighteenth century and spread with great rapidity as the pioneers moved westward. There have been severe outbreaks at various times among the horses and mules of the United States Army, and the Army was charged with introducing the infection into Mexico during the Mexican War. Before the disease was brought under control by improved sanitary measures and reliable diagnostic tests at the beginning of the present century, any concentration of horses and mules, particularly in the, larger cities, was a fertile field for glanders.

At the present time the occurrence of glanders in the United States is almost negligible. For this reason the precautions being taken by the Department of Agriculture to guard against its reintroduction from abroad through careful supervision, including veterinary inspection at designated ports of entry of all importations of susceptible animals, are of great importance, though this is probably not fully appreciated except by those closely connected with the importation of equines.

Symptoms and Lesions

The period of incubation, or the time elapsing between the exposure to infection and the appearance of recognized symptoms, may vary from a few days to several months, but under natural conditions it averages about 2 weeks. The disease assumes either on acute or a chronic form. Asses and mules, as a general rule, manifest the acute symptoms, which progress rapidly, whereas horses almost invariably have the chronic or slowly developing type.

For convenient description the principal symptoms and lesions of typical cases may be classified as nasal, pulmonary, and cutaneous. It should be understood, however, that these forms may occur simultaneously.

Nasal Form

The first symptom likely to be noticed is a nasal mucous discharge in one or more rarely, both nostrils, which later becomes copious and purulent (full of pus). Examination of the mucous membrane of the nasal cavity in the early stages should disclose numerous nodules, ranging from the size of bird shot to that of a pea, which are red and quite firm to the touch. These soon break down into ragged-edged ulcers which pour forth a viscous, sticky material, yellowish in color except for an occasional trace of blood. This condition is often present on the membranous covering of the larynx and trachea. When healing takes place the ulcers are replaced by characteristic radiating or star-shaped scar tissue. These symptoms are associated with enlargement of the submaxillary glands under the lower jaw toward the throat, which become indurated, or hardened, as in the acute form of strangles. The condition differs from strangles in that the glands rarely abscess and erupt.

Pulmonary Form

The most constant seat of glanderous lesions is the lungs. Seldom If ever are these organs wholly sound when there is clinical evidence of the disease elsewhere in the body. Attention may be attracted first to the animal's loss of condition and lack of endurance when worked and the sudden bleeding of the nose from destructive pulmonary processes. Painful spasmodic coughing and the resultant dislodgment of a thick mucus discharge from the nostrils very definitely point to lung involvement. In the early stages of typical cases, firm nodules ranging from the size of a small pea to that of a hen's egg may be found embedded in otherwise healthy-appearing lung tissue. At first dark red and slightly translucent, these nodules gradually take on a whitish, opaque appearance. As the disease progresses the affected lung tissue becomes dark red owing to the presence of excess blood, and in later stages areas containing caseous, or cheese-like, masses are in evidence. The lymph glands of the thoracic (chest) cavity become enlarged and develop nodular lesions similar to those occurring in the lungs.

Cutaneous Form

The development of nodules and ulcers in the skin and subcutaneous tissue is a common occurrence in glanders. This is the form which is often referred to as farcy. In the skin proper the nodules, which are about the size of a pea, soon break down to form ulcers. The deeper lying indurated nodules of the subcutaneous tissue (beneath the skin), usually on the limbs, chest, and lower abdomen, may reach the size of a walnut. These also disintegrate into ulcers, which are much deeper than those in the skin and exude a purulent material streaked with blood. Upon healing, the ulcers leave radiating scar tissue. The lymphatic vessels in the region of the nodules and ulcers become thickened and stand out like cords. In the meanwhile a painless swelling, or subcutaneous edema, occurs on the under side of the abdomen and chest and may extend down the limbs, becoming a serious impediment to walking.

Diagnosis and Treatment

The micro-organism responsible for glanders, *Bacillus mallei*, possesses no characteristics by which it may be readily distinguished from many other bacteria that may be present in glanderous discharges. This greatly limits the possibility of making a diagnosis by microscopic examination. Fortunately, reliable diagnosis may be made by use of the mallein test, the serum test, or animal inoculation. The mallein test is made by observing the results of the introduction into the eye of a few drops of a product derived from cultures of the causative organism. This test is the one most commonly used because of the simplicity of its application and its reliability in detecting all forms, including latent cases, with sufficient accuracy to accomplish complete eradication of the disease when followed by proper sanitary measures.

Since the discovery of mallein as a diagnostic agent for glanders, numerous experiments have been conducted to ascertain whether it has any immunizing or curative value. All attempts to build up immunity against glanders in susceptible animals by vaccination have failed. Spontaneous recovery sometimes occurs, but it does not confer immunity against subsequent infection. For this reason treatment of affected animals with either medicines or biological products is not recommended as a means of controlling outbreaks.

Methods of Eradication

In glanderous equines the causative organism is excreted in large numbers from lesions of the skin, lungs, and respiratory tract. Therefore objects likely to be contaminated with these pus-laden excretions are to be looked upon as especially dangerous in the spread of the disease. Water troughs, pails, feed, mangers, bedding, harness, grooming, utensils, and other objects become important factors in transmitting the disease from infected to healthy animals. The reservoir for the infection is the diseased animal, which rarely recovers. Consequently, animals presenting symptoms resembling those of glanders should be isolated and mallein-tested by a qualified veterinarian. If the test shows that the disease is present, the animal should be destroyed without delay and the exposed premises and equipment thoroughly cleaned and disinfected. The usual procedure in eradicating the disease is to hold all susceptible animals in the community under strict sanitary control until the diagnostic test has been applied to those even remotely exposed and all reactors among them have been disposed of in a safe manner.

Many of the States have laws and regulations which require the prompt reporting of suspected cases of glanders and provide for the payment of indemnity for animals destroyed under official direction.

Chapter 5

DOURINE

T.W. Cole[1]

[1] *T.W. Cole is Assistant Chief, Field Inspection Division, Bureau of Animal Industry.*

A dangerous disease of horses and other equines, dourine is similar to syphilis in human beings. Early diagnosis of dourine, by a serum test, has contributed greatly to progress in eradicating the disease.

Dourine, an Arabic word meaning unclean, denotes a specific infectious disease transmitted from animal to animal almost exclusively by copulation. The disease is also known by a number of other names such as "maladie du coit," "equine syphilis," "genital glanders," and "breeding paralysis." It is contracted under normal conditions only by the horse and ass. The causative organism, *Trypanosoma equiperdum*, is an animal parasite of microscopic size.

History

That dourine had entered the United States was first definitely recognized in 1886, when an outbreak occurred in the vicinity of Bloomington, Ill., as a result of the importation of a stallion from France for breeding purposes. Rigid control measures were put into effect promptly by State officials after the disease was diagnosed. Unfortunately, prior to official recognition of the disease, infected animals had been moved out of the district, and these no doubt set up new centers of infection. At any rate, after the initial outbreak the disease was detected at irregular intervals in Nebraska and South

Dakota, but it was finally brought under control, In 1906, however, a new center of infection developed in Iowa. Despite the energetic measures adopted by both State and Federal authorities, this outbreak was not curbed until 1911.

The greatest early handicap in combating dourine was the lack of any diagnostic test. In 1912 the complement-fixation blood-serum test, requiring special laboratory facilities and the services of a trained bacteriologist, was perfected. Its use in testing horses imported from countries in which dourine is present has been an important aid in guarding against further introduction of the disease from abroad. Through this test dourine has been found over a large area in the West, including Iowa, North Dakota., South Dakota, Nebraska, Colorado, Wyoming, Montana, Idaho, Oregon, California, Nevada, Arizona, and New Mexico. Notable success has been attained in its eradication, and at present (January 1942) the only known areas of infection remaining are in Arizona, California, and Nevada.

Symptoms

The symptoms vary in individual horses and usually appear in two distinct stages. In the first the sexual organs are affected principally, but if the disease progresses into the second or a later chronic; stage, nervous disorders become pronounced. The period of incubation, or time elapsing before clinical symptoms appear after exposure to infection, ranges from 8 days to 2 months. At times the initial symptoms are slight and may escape unobserved unless dourine is known to exist in the vicinity.

In the stallion the disease usually begins with a swelling of the prepuce, or sheath, a condition which later spreads forward to the abdomen and backward to the scrotum. If the inflammation extends to the testicles, these parts become enlarged and sensitive to pressure. During this time usually the penis is constantly affected and partially protrudes from its sheath, swollen and discharging a yellowish fluid from the urethra. Small blisters, or vesicles that appear on the penis and sheath in the early stages soon rupture and form raw, irregular ulcers, singly and in groups. These ulcers heal, leaving permanent white scars which are highly significant in diagnosing the disease by physical examination. While the symptoms are developing, the stallion manifests a repeated desire to urinate, and the breeding instinct is intensified until frequently it becomes inordinate.

In mares the early symptoms are swollen external genitals, causing a gaping vulva which exposes the clitoris in a constant state of erection. Swelling may also occur in the region of the mammary glands. Early symptoms may include manifestations of uneasiness–switching of the tail and frequent voiding of small quantities of urine–resembling prolonged heat. A scant or copious discharge similar to that found in the stallion may be present. Vesicles, or blisters, which appear on the inner mucous membrane and outer skin of the genitals soon rupture, leaving deep-seated ulcers that, when healed, form rather prominent white scars, distinguished by their permanency from the temporary ones produced by other affections, such as coital exanthema.

The second stage of dourine in animals of both sexes is marked by nervous or constitutional disturbances that may not appear for months or even years after the acute symptoms subside. The cutaneous, or skin, lesions, which are essentially secondary, follow the symptoms in the genital organs and appear in the form of urticarial wheals or plaques resembling those in hives. These are highly characteristic. They vary from the size of a dime to that of a dollar or larger and may be round or irregular in form. The wheals are produced by infiltration of serum into the papillary (hair-producing) layer of the skin and cause the hair to stand erect. The commonest locations of these lesions are on the chest, belly, and croup, but they may appear on the neck, shoulders, withers, or other parts of the body. After these small raised areas subside, the skin is not infrequently left depigmented or covered with white hair.

The advanced cases of dourine are characterized by loss of flesh, nervousness, and paralysis. At times the nerves of the face are affected, causing paralysis of one ear, an eyelid, a nostril, or a lip, or of one whole side of the face. However, paralysis most commonly affects the hind legs, causing the animal to stub or drag a toe in walking, with a tendency to knuckling. When paralysis of the hindquarters occurs, the disease usually progresses rapidly. Muscles become weakened and atrophied until the animal can no longer stand, and it goes down and dies in a state of nervous exhaustion.

Treatment

Efforts to protect animals by immunization or to develop a satisfactory medicinal treatment for dourine have been disappointing. Unsatisfactory results from lines of treatment found useful in combating other trypanosome infections are apparently due to the failure of drugs to reach and destroy all the causative organisms. Those located in edematous swellings joint cavities, and other parts of the body escape and give rise to relapses.

Recovery from dourine is always uncertain. A mortality of 50 percent is not uncommon, and in some outbreaks in other countries losses of as many as 70 percent of the animals affected have been reported when the disease was permitted to run its course. Infected mares seldom conceive, and those that do are likely to abort. Affected stallions are usually reservoirs of infection and may spread the disease with great rapidity over large areas. In this country, where the disease has existed only in restricted areas; sanitary conditions demand its eradication.

Methods of Eradication

Dourine is spread under natural conditions only by the act of coition. Any sanitary measures for its eradication must necessarily include a ban on the breeding of infected animals. An occasional animal may apparently recover, but it remains a potential spreader, for very often infection is present in a dormant state and the excitement of copulation tends to cause its reappearance with renewed vigor. Spaying mares and castrating stallions, especially under range conditions, where the disease has occurred most frequently in the United States, is a temporizing method of control such mares may be covered by a stallion, and even after castration infected stallions may spread the disease to healthy mares. The most effective method of eradicating the disease is the prompt destruction of in infected animals.

The Pathological Division of the Bureau of Animal Industry maintains a diagnostic laboratory in Washington, D.C., properly equipped to apply the complement-fixation test for dourine when samples of blood serum are submitted for examination. Preparing serum samples for the test requires skip and experience and should be undertaken only by a qualified veterinarian.

The Bureau of Animal Industry also cooperates with livestock sanitary authorities in dealing with dourine in the field wherever it exists. In this work animals are held under strict surveillance until the results of tests are knows and those found harboring infection are promptly destroyed. The usual procedure is for the state and Federal Governments to share equally in the expense of indemnifying the owners for animals destroyed, except on Indian reservations, where the entire expense is borne by the Federal Government (Fig. 1). In the eradication programmes, animals whose serum gives negative results are classed as free from the disease and released for breeding.

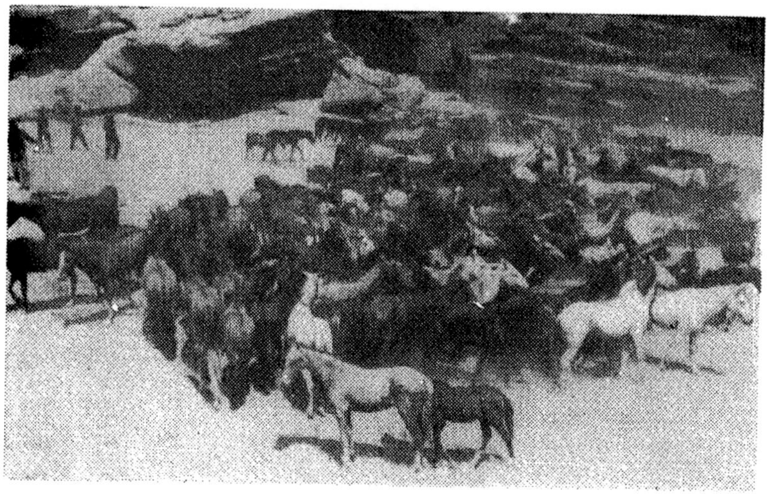

Fig. 1: Wild range horses that have been brought to an enclosure so that they may be tested for dourine. In testing, a blood sample is taken from each animal of breeding age.

Chapter 6

MISCELLANEOUS DISEASES OF EQUINES

L.O. Mott, M.S. Shahan, L.T. Giltner & A.H. Frank[1]

[1] *L.O. Mott is Assistant Veterinarian, M.S. Shahan is Veterinarian, and L.T. Giltner is Senior Veterinarian, Pathological Division and A.H. Frank is Assistant Veterinarian, Animal Disease Station, Beltsville, Md., Bureau of Animal Industry.*

Here are facts, particularly from the standpoint of symptoms, causes, treatment, and prevention, about a large number of diseases of horses and mules.

Influenza

Equine influenza, also known as shipping fever, pinkeye, catarrhal fever, epizootic cellulitis, and, among older horsemen, epizooty, is probably the most contagious and widely distributed disease to which horses, mules, and asses are susceptible. The death rate, though sometimes as high as 10 percent of the cases, is not so great as that from some other infectious diseases, but the economic loss entailed by the incapacity of affected animals for work is in the aggregate serious.

Horses and mules coming through sales stables, stockyards, remount depots, and other establishments where large numbers of animals from scattered sources are held together for some time are especially apt to develop influenza. The symptoms are strikingly like those of influenza in man or similar conditions in other species although there is no proved connection.

Fever (103°-106°F.),[2] extreme weakness and depression, rapid breathing, harsh cough, and watery discharges from the nostrils and eyes are common early indications of the infection. The conjunctiva, the lining membrane of the eyelid, becomes yellowish pink in color (so-called pinkeye). Swelling due to edema (accumulations of the watery constituents of the blood and lymph) of the legs, abdomen, and head are common symptoms in many outbreaks. The affected animal stands in an attitude of extreme dejection, drinks eagerly but sparingly, and eats little, in some cases finally refusing feed altogether. Sometimes there is restlessness and continuous shifting of weight from one leg to another, with a cracking sound in the joints.

In uncomplicated cases the temperature returns to normal within a week and gradual recovery follows. On the other hand, a second rise in temperature, often fluctuating, may occur, ushering in more or less serious complications, such as pneumonia, with rapid, labored breathing; inflammation of the stomach and intestines, usually with constipation and later a profuse, fetid diarrhoea; inflammation of the kidneys, as usually indicated by frequent but scanty urination; inflammation of the brain, as shown by symptoms of paralysis or twitching and nervous excitability; abscess formation in the lymph nodes of the body, especially about the head (commonly referred to as strangles); and even degeneration of the heart muscle), with serious changes in the character and rate of the pulse. Severe swellings about the eyes may occur, and sometimes even blindness results.

This disease, like influenza of man and of swine, is caused primarily by a filterable virus, complications being attributable to miscellaneous bacteria, chiefly streptococci. Excessive hard work, undue exposure, and generally poor hygienic conditions are contributory factors. Symptoms develop as early as 3 days or as late as 2 weeks after exposure.

Prevention and Treatment

Horses and mules being brought on to the farm or into the stable from outside sources, especially sales establishments, stockyards,

---

[2] The normal temperature of the horse is 99.5°-100.5° F.

or remount depots, should be held in rigid quarantine, isolated in a separate stable with separate attendants, for 10 to 30 days.

Animals going to market can apparently be protected to some degree by the repeated injection of bacterins, prepared from killed cultures of the bacteria commonly found as so-called secondary invaders in the disease.

Some apparently fully recovered animals may harbor the virus in the blood stream or, in the case of stallions, in the semen, for months and thus be a source of infection of other animals.

The first symptoms of the disease in an animal should immediately lead to its isolation and a thorough cleaning and disinfection of the stable, including troughs, feed boxes, buckets, etc. Although the disease is highly contagious, its spread may be much lessened by promptness in these matters.

Experiments with the object of perfecting a vaccine for prevention and a serum for treatment of Influenza are being carried out. So far no specific biological or chemical preventive or cure is available.

The first principle of treatment is absolute rest for the affected animal at the first signs of illness. He should be placed in a freshly bedded, well-ventilated but draft-free stall, and provided with small amounts of nutritious but not heavy feed. Fresh, clean water should be kept before him. It may be advisable to keep him blanketed, but this should not prevent regular grooming.

Such medicinal treatment as is given should be restricted to that, specifically prescribed by the veterinarian. This may include inhalation of medicated vapor, medicines to regulate the bowels, stimulants, etc. In some cases it may be necessary to feed the animal artificially. This is usually done by introducing feed into the stomach by means of the stomach tube, or it may be introduced rectally. Blood or blood serum from recovered cases may be administered.

Animals should not be returned to work until some days after the temperature has become normal and full strength has returne.

Distemper (Strangles)

In past years when traffic in horses and mules was heavy and these animals were used by practically all farmers to haul farm produce and for transportation, equine distemper was widespread and common in the United States. Animals from the countryside came in contact with city delivery horses on streets, in public stables, and at public watering troughs. It was an exceptional horse or mule that reached the age of 5 years without exposure to the infection, and practically every one developed the disease.

Today, there are large numbers of horses on isolated farms that have never been exposed to the infection and are consequently as susceptible as the colts of the previous era. The disease persists to a greater or less extent in stockyards, sales stables, race tracks, and remount depots. Practically every animal held in such places for any length of time is exposed to distemper, as well as to influenza. When a horse or mule is taken from a point of heavy concentration of animals from diverse sources to an isolated farm or breeding stable, the possibility of the infection being carried along is great.

The essential cause of the disease is generally conceded to be the germ known as *Streptococcus equi*, an organism which is easily spread from an affected animal either directly or indirectly by way of watering troughs, feed boxes, mangers, blankets, halters, etc., as well as on the person of the attendant. Cold, poorly ventilated stables, undue exposure to severe weather, and overwork are contributing influences, and the disease is most prevalent during the spring months. The disease affects only solipeds (horses, mules, and asses). Recovered animals generally remain immune for the rest of their lives, except in rare cases when they are exposed to an extremely virulent form of the disease. The main detrimental effects to owners are impairment in the development of colts and loss of the services of working animals, but in some outbreaks the disease may be fatal in as many as 5 percent of the cases.

The onset of the disease is sudden, usually within 3 to 8 days after exposure. The early symptoms are somewhat like those of influenza. There is fever (104°-106°F.), reduced appetite, and great depression. The membranes of the nose become red and dry, and a watery discharge from the nostrils follows. After 1 to 3 days, the discharge becomes very thick and profuse and is expelled in great quantities by snorting or coughing. In a majority of cases there is a hot, painful swelling of the lymph glands (submaxillary) under the lower jaw near the threat. These frequently become abscessed, and a yellow, creamy pus is formed. In uncomplicated cases, the fever drops, appetite returns, and the spirit revives shortly after the abscesses are drained, through either spontaneous rupture or surgical drainage, the disease lasting 2 to 4 weeks.

Complications are common, however, and abscesses may form in other lymph glands in the body, even in the abdominal cavity. Abscesses in the deeper glands and other tissues of the head and throat often obstruct the breathing, and it may be necessary to place a tube in the trachea (windpipe) to avoid suffocation. Pneumonia may result from spread of the infection, often through the inhalation of pus from ruptured glands. Septicemia, or so-called blood poisoning, not infrequently occurs.

The mortality may be high in young foals, which sometimes contract the disease, and in newborn foals, which may be born with the infection.

Treatment and Prevention

The first provision for an animal affected with distemper should be its immediate isolation from other animals in a clean, well-bedded, draft-free stall. All equipment with which it has been in contact should be thoroughly cleaned and disinfected. All discharges, bedding, and excreta from sick animals should be burned or buried.

Complete rest, a constant supply of pure, clean water and a moderate amount of nutritious, laxative feed should be provided. The fact that mild, sporadic cases often require no further treatment explains the apparent efficacy of many home-compounded and proprietary medicines advertised as specific cures for the disease. As a matter of fact there is no such medicine for strangles. Veterinary attention is, however, frequently desirable and necessary.

As mentioned before, it may be necessary to place a tube in the trachea to prevent suffocation. Lancing the abscesses may be advisable. Medicines designed to aid the discharge of excessive secretions in the air passages are frequently prescribed. Medicated vapors are sometimes used as inhalants. Cloths soaked in hot liquids are frequently applied to the swollen glands. Blood or blood serum from recovered cases is sometimes employed. Stimulants may be indicated.

For the prevention of the disease, a bacterin prepared from cultures of the germs found in cases of the disease is sometimes used. For best results, repeated doses should be given prior to anticipated possible exposure such as could be encountered in the course of shipping or at shows or race meetings. The precaution of quarantining newly purchased animals in a separate, isolated stable for 2 to 4 weeks before allowing contact with the "home" animals is very desirable.

Purpura Hemorrhagica (Petechial Fever)

Purpura hemorrhagica is a noncontagious affection which commonly follows severe or complicated cases of other diseases of equines, especially influenza and distemper. While the essential cause is unknown, it rarely occurs except after a severe septic infection.

The malady is generally attributed to a decrease in the thrombocytes or platelets (cellular constituents of the blood concerned with clotting) resulting from the presence of poisonous chemical substances in the blood. It occurs in some cases of fistula or poll evil or subsequent to the development of an abscess or of necrosis (death of tissue) anywhere in the body. Sometimes it appears without a known history, of any such process. Rarely more than one or at most a few animals, in a stable develop the disease. It usually occurs in the spring or early summer following epizootics (outbreaks) of other diseases. Animals under 2 years of age are seldom affected.

The disease is characterized by hemorrhages and edema in the, skin, inner membranes, muscle, internal organs, and other tissues of the body. In some particulars the symptoms are somewhat suggestive of swamp fever (equine infectious anemia). The disease usually begins with hemorrhages in the nasal membranes. Later, swellings appear about the lips, eyelids, legs, or lower part of the abdomen. The swellings are cold and painless, usually sharply outlined but sometimes diffuse, invariably pitting under pressure. They may appear suddenly or develop gradually during several days.

The temperature is usually normal or only slightly increased (102°-103° F.), but the pulse is quickened materially. The membranes at the body openings frequently become yellowish in color (icterus, or jaundice). The average course of the disease is 12 to 15 days, but this is variable, and recurrence of the trouble is not uncommon, especially if the animal is worked or vigorously exercised.

Complications are common. Among these are pneumonia, severe inflammations of the stomach or intestines, and severe anemia (deficiency of blood and of red blood cells). All may lead to a prolonged serious illness and death.

In addition to complete rest, hygienic stabling conditions, and reasonable feeding, treatment is directed toward the alleviation of certain symptoms as they develop or can be anticipated in individual cases. Insertion of a trachea tube to facilitate breathing and the use of stimulants are sometimes advisable. The unrestricted use of purgatives is believed to be harmful in most cases. Direct transfusions of blood are commonly employed. Certain drugs are injected into the blood stream by some veterinarians as a part of the treatment.

Wounds and Wound Infections

Of all domestic animals the horse is most subject to accidental wounds. Moreover, it is more susceptible to infections than other domestic animals, especially in wounds that are neglected or unwisely handled. Mules are definitely less likely than horses to acquire accidental wounds, but when they do, infection is a potential hazard.

Many of the germs that commonly result in serious trouble are widely distributed in the soil and in forage or manure. Among them are those of the genus *Clostridiwm*, including *Clostridium septicum*, which is the cause of various types of so-called gas gangrene and malignant edema, and *Clostridium tetani*, the organism that causes tetanus, or lockjaw. These belong to the class of germs known as anaerobes, which thrive in the absence of air. When implanted in injured tissues from which the air is excluded by surface healing or improper dressings, they become especially active and dangerous. Also, they form a spore, or seed form, which is capable of growth even after doing for years outside of an animal body. Such germs as streptococci, staphylococci, and some bacteria in the class known as aerobes, which implies their need for air for best growth, are especially apt to cause the formation of pus. In addition to the so-called pure infections induced by a single type of germ, mixed infections involving more than one type may occur.

The skin has the function of assisting in the elimination of body wastes through sweating and also acts as a protective covering for the body. But it is a basic fact that the skin of an animal is never free from germs, some of which are often of a type capable of causing serious trouble. When the skin is broken by a cut, bruise, or even superficial chafing, access to the inner tissues is open to germs from the hair and skin surface or the injuring object. The sound body reacting normally usually overcomes the threatened invasion. But if the resistance of the body tissues is low, if severe injury occurs, or if the germs are especially numerous or virulent in character, infection follows as a matter of course.

The resistance of the animal's body or the character and number of the germs may be such as to result in the confinement of the trouble to the region where the germs gain entrance. In such a localized infection, there will be redness, swelling, and more or less pain, with or without the formation of gas or pus. But if the army of invading organisms succeeds in overcoming the protective forces called into action by the body, a general or systemic infection, known as septicemia or pyemia (blood poisoning), results, and in addition to the local indications, fever, depression, stiffness, loss of appetite, and other evidences of the spread of the germs in the blood occur. Death of the affected animal is common, especially if treatment is not promptly instituted.

Tetanus is caused by a powerful toxin, or poison, formed in the body by the specific germ of the disease, *Clostridium tetani*. Practically all animals, including man, are susceptible, the horse, mule, and ass being especially so. Symptoms of tetanus appear in the majority of causes in 1 to 2 weeks after the germs gain entrance to the body, or they may be delayed for months, according to the severity of the primary injury and the degree of infection. On the other hand, young animals especially may develop symptoms in less than a week.

The first signs of the disease are usually observed about the head. Chewing is less forceful than normal, and swallowing is slow and awkward. The nictitating membrane (the so-called inner or third eyelid between the lower eyelid and the eyeball proper) protrudes up on the surface of the eyeball. The rigidity of the muscles due to spasm spreads, sometimes rapidly, from one group of muscles to another. Eating is greatly impaired or even completely prevented (lockjaw), the legs are spread and stiffened, giving the appearance of a sawhorse, the tail is elevated and stiff, and the ears are held rigidly erect. Constipation commonly occurs. The breathing is rapid and forced the heart action mayor may not be quickened, and usually there is little if any fever except in the severe cases, and then near death. The muscles may tend to relax at intervals, only to contract instantly, with the rapidity of a spring, at the slightest noise, a ray of light, or a touch on the body. Death is usually due to sheer exhaustion, paralysis of the vital organs, or pneumonia resulting from inhaling feed, throat secretions, or medicines which have been improperly administered. Animals which recover are often sick for a month or more.

Prevention and Treatment

Localized wound infections, septicemia, pyemia, and tetanus are largely preventable. In the first place, sharp objects should not be allowed in the stables, corrals, paddocks, or pastures used by horses. Barbed-wire fencing should be replaced by board or pole fences. Trees and shrubs should be trimmed at intervals, broken or low-hanging limbs being removed. Farm machinery should not remain in the barnyard or field where horses may be free. Scrap metal, wire, boards, nails, etc., should be kept away from all kinds of livestock as well as horses. Loose nails, screws, hinges, and door fasteners, splintered boards, and other sharp protruding objects should not be permitted in stables or elsewhere where horses are kept.

Quietness and gentleness are especially desirable attributes in stable workers. General cleanliness and hygiene will lessen infections when injuries occur. In some sections tetanus is especially prevalent, so much so that even surgical operations such as must be performed in the stable or barnyard may predispose an animal to the disease. Some truck gardens, heavily manured lands, and swamps are hotbeds for the tetanus organism and its spores. In such locations, the use of tetanus antitoxin in the form of serum is good insurance against the disease in case of any injury to animals, especially horses. Tetanus toxoid, the chemically treated toxin produced by the germ of tetanus, engenders a strong long-standing immunity against the disease. It is employed as a routine matter in some armies and may be advisedly used in certain localities where the disease is commonly prevalent.

The treatment to be used for wounds depends upon the location and extent of the injury and the likelihood of infection. The majority of wounds, although potentially dangerous, do best if left entirely alone awaiting direct attention by the veterinarian. This does not apply in all cases, of course, as, for example, where the injury has caused profuse bleeding. Blood flowing through and over injured tissue in a moderate amount is a natural and desirable development in a wound. The loss of 1 to 2 quarts or even more blood by a robust horse or mule is not in itself dangerous, but if bleeding is long continued, severe weakening or even death may result. In serious cases it may be possible to stop the flow of blood by the direct application of pressure over the part with a pad of sterile gauze or other suitable material. If this fails, and the wound is on a leg or other part to which a tourniquet may be applied, one may be adjusted above the injury. This may be done simply by passing a thick twisted cloth about the leg and tying it loosely. A stick is then inserted in the space between the cloth and the leg and twisted to a degree of tightness sufficient to lessen or stop the bleeding. The tourniquet must not be applied too tightly, and it should be loosened every 20 minutes so that the blood flow beyond the wound is not cut off entirely. Such substances as flour or earth should never be placed in a wound to stop bleeding, nor should turpentine, crude creosote products, or other irritating substances be used as antiseptics.

To avoid further injury it may be necessary to withdraw an object extending into the wound, but care must be taken not to break it off, leaving a fragment deeply embedded in the tissues. Further possible injury and infection should be avoided by confining the animal in clean quarters.

Upon his arrival, the veterinarian first surveys the damage. Then bleeding vessels are picked up by forceps and tied with a suitable ligature. It is usually desirable to clean the skin in the vicinity of the wound, care being taken that the materials used do not drip or run into the wound. Hair, straw, and other foreign materials are picked from the wound with sterile forceps, the hand or fingers never touching the wound directly. Unless exceptionally heavy contamination of the wound has occurred, strong antiseptic solutions are seldom desirable or necessary. Rather, mild substances, such as physiological salt solution (having the same salt content as the body tissues) which may be made by adding 1 teaspoonful of common table salt to 1 pint of boiled water, are used to sponge the exposed surfaces of the wound lightly. If the wound is relatively clean and not too extensive or gaping, the muscles and skin may be drawn together by sutures. Some wounds heal better without any bandage; a bandage serves to protect others against further infection or to support the tissues. A heavy bandage serves in some cases to keep various dressing compounds in contact with the wound. In severe, contused wounds, examinations are made for fractures of the underlying bones.

Many neglected wounds of the foot that do not result in immediate lameness may cause extreme lameness some days later through the damming up of inflammatory wound secretions or pus. The sole of the hoof must often be deeply pared away before the site of the wound is discovered. The area of discoloration must then be enlarged to permit the escape of the material resulting from the infection and the application of antiseptic substances. In areas where tetanus is prevalent, such wounds are especially conducive to that disease.

The treatment of tetanus is often not entirely satisfactory; yet occasional cases eventually recover without any treatment. It is first desirable to open the wound through which the infection entered, if this can be located, thoroughly draining it and applying suitable antiseptics. Confinement in a clean, cool, quiet, darkened stall with as little disturbance as possible is advantageous. If tetanus antitoxin is given–and its use is merited for especially valuable animals and in other selected cases–huge and often repeated dosing is usually required. Further, sedatives of various types are commonly employed, and artificial feeding may be required.

Slight wounds or simple abrasions of the skin, if immediately treated with fresh tincture of iodine U.S.P., seldom cause trouble except in tetanus districts.

Wounds in which foreign material is allowed to remain or which are otherwise neglected commonly develop pus, for the elimination of which surgical incision, drainage, and repeated irrigation with antiseptics may be required.

Horses obliged to lean heavily on a high manger or other fixture to obtain feed frequently develop an accumulation of serum (the watery constituent of blood and lymph) in the breast tissues. Successful treatment of these formations, which are usually free from bacteria, commonly requires incision, drainage, and irrigation or packing.

Chronically inflamed wounds, such as wire cuts, sometimes develop excessive scar tissue, known as keloid. Surgical removal is the only generally applicable treatment for such cases.

Breeding Troubles

The broad scope of the term "breeding troubles" is apparent when it is considered that it includes any cause of barrenness in either the mare or the stallion and the abnormal termination of pregnancy in abortions and stillbirths, as well as the problems of foaling. The importance of proper care and management of breeding animals is well emphasized by the vast amount of literature available to the farmer and the breeder in the form of bulletins and farm and breed magazines. Yet, despite this available information, in too many instances the possible generous margin of profit from horse and mule husbandry under normal conditions is lost through careless or ignorant handling of breeding animals. The method of handling animals has a decided influence on their physical condition and health. In normal, healthy individuals, the husbandman can prevent an over-nourished or undernourished condition and provide proper exercise, which with good housing and sanitation will do more than anything else to prevent breeding troubles. Regardless of the success of preventive measures, however, he cannot by these methods alone control all the physiological upsets or the invasion of all the diseases which affect sexual activities.

Anatomy and Physiology

The anatomy and physiology of the genital organs of the mare are very complex. Briefly, the genital tract begins at the external opening, known as the vulva, which opens forward into the vagina. The vagina leads into the uterus (womb) through a narrow, thick-walled neck, or cervix. The uterus branches into two so-called horns. Attached to each of these there is a fine tube, the Fallopian tube, designed to convey the egg from the ovary into the uterus, where it is fertilized by one of the multitudinous sperm cells from the male.

The sexual behavior of normal animals is controlled by secretions (hormones) from certain body glands, as discussed elsewhere in this volume.

An upset in the secretion of any of the primary sex hormones may produce sterility in either sex. In the female it may interrupt the coordinated sexual rhythm, prevent conception, or induce early or late abortion. Its effect on the male may be manifested by impotency or sluggish activity and sterility. Much has been accomplished in the treatment of glandular deficiency by proper diagnosis and by the administration of the hormone indicated.

Normally, the egg is expelled from the ovary of the mare close to the end of estrus (about 24 or 48 hours before the end of heat) and is capable of becoming fertilized for only about 12 to 24 hours afterward. The spermatozoa live for about 12 to 48 hours in the genital tract of the mare, the time varying with individual stallions. If the sperm of a given stallion is capable of living only about 12 hours, more frequent matings would be necessary in order to obtain a rate of fertility equal to that of a stallion whose sperm would live an average of 48 hours. These facts show the desirability of breeding the mare 1 to 2 days before she goes out of heat. There is no method, except by individual records, to determine the length of the estrus period. In the absence of such records, in order to breed at the proper time one would have to breed a mare every other day through each estrus period in order to insure pregnancy.

Efficiently kept breeding records and observations on fertile animals indicate that the selection of a particular day for breeding during the period of estrus may largely determine the chances of conception. Estrus has been found to vary in duration from 2 to 30 days in different individuals. However, the periods for an individual mare seldom vary in length by more than 1 to 2 days, so they are of sufficient regularity that records can be relied upon for selection of the proper time for mating.

Breeding Hygiene

The success of many large, privately owned breeding establishments and Army remount breeding stations must be attributed largely to careful examination and selection of prospective breeding animals, as well as to breeding hygiene. The complete programme is quite elaborate, but the basic principles can be given briefly.

To begin with, each mare and stallion is chosen on the basis of suitable ancestry and acceptable conformation as individuals. The animals must be free of transmissible disease, and the genitalia must be normal.

The mares to be bred are examined during an interval between periods of heat to determine that there is no inflammation of the genital tract. The presence of infection may sometimes but not always be indicated by a discharge from the vulva. Consequently, close examination is required.

After the hind parts of the mare have been thoroughly washed with clean, warm water and a mild soap and dried, the veterinarian inspects the vagina and cervix for the presence of infection by the use of a speculum and light. Infection is usually readily recognized from the appearance of the structures and the character of the secretions, but it may be necessary or desirable to obtain a specimen for laboratory examination.

A manual examination is also made of the ovaries and uterus through the walls of the rectum. The presence of large cysts or excessive fibrous tissue in the ovaries, conditions likely to preclude conception, is thus discovered. Such conditions may be corrected by manual treatment or by the use of hormones, but they are sometimes incurable.

If evidence of infection is discovered in the genital organs, the mare is withheld from breeding until the organs become normal. If the mare is bred while the organs are infected failure to conceive is common, or if the mare does become pregnant, abortion or the delivery of a weak, infected foal may follow.

Mares are also examined after foaling. The genital organs should return to normal within 8 days, and mares normally come into heat in 7 to 12 days. They may be examined on the sixth or seventh day and if found normal may be bred at this early heat. Many large breeding establishments make it a practice not to breed at this time but to wait until the second heat period. Much future trouble, such as infections and abortions, may be avoided by this practice.

The serviceability of the stallion is checked at intervals by microscopic examination and bacteriological cultures of the semen. An infected stallion is not permitted to serve mares, especially clean ones.

The correction of genital infections in mares is, strictly speaking, a veterinarian's task. It is not to be undertaken by a layman through such practices as promiscuous douching and "opening the womb." Some mares become infected by the free entrance of air and foreign matter into the vagina between the lips of a flaccid or gaping vulva. In such cases, the lips are frequently sutured or clipped together along the upper part of the vulva. After healing, the sutures or clips are removed. Such treatment in the fall usually leads to good breeding condition by the following spring. At mating, care must be taken that the closed portion of the vulva is not torn. At foaling time the adhesions are broken down to permit free passage of the foal.

Service

Estrus, or heat, in most cases is determined by teasing the mare with a stallion. One familiar with the habits of horses can determine whether or not the mare will accept the stallion. Some mares, however, do not show outward signs of heat and remain indifferent when brought in contact with the stallion. Heat may also be determined by a vaginal examination with the speculum. Some mares come into heat at very irregular intervals, in extreme cases only every other year. Hormonal treatment may be indicated for such mares.

In preparation for service, or breeding, the external genital organs of the mare are prepared as for vaginal examination, and in addition the tail may be wrapped with a sterile bandage. The stallion should have a similar cleansing, both before and after service, time being taken to remove all sebum adhering to the penis. Careful technique at this time may prevent the introduction of infection into the mare.

There are two methods used to breed mares–normal mating to a stallion or jack and artificial insemination. In either case extreme hygienic precautions should be observed.

After normal mating, as the stallion dismounts, a portion of semen is generally discharged from the penis. A container may be held under the penis to collect the semen for examination.

If artificial insemination is practiced, the stallion is cleansed as for service and allowed to mount a mare and ejaculate into a sterile artificial vagina which is held to one side of the mare at an angle near the vagina. This method has many advantages over normal matings. The semen can be examined to determine its quality before use. A sample may be stored for some time, transported for considerable distances, and divided for the insemination of several mares. The spread of venereal diseases may thus be prevented, and samples may be examined for the presence of infection.

Diagnosis of Pregnancy

Pregnancy can be readily diagnosed by an experienced veterinarian by manual examination within a few months after conception. Pregnancy may also be determined between the forty-second and one hundred and twentieth days after conception by the injection of blood serum from the mare into female rabbits or young rats or mice. During this period the pregnant mare's serum contains s a hormone which, when injected into the test animals, causes activation of the ovary and enlargement of the uterus. Observations of these changes may be made through operation on the rabbit, which may be used over and over again, and in rats and mice after the animals are killed.

Abortion

Of all mares that become pregnant, it is estimated that two-thirds will have normal healthy foals and one-third will either abort or produce a weak, infected foal. Under optimum conditions in a given stable, however, the losses should be negligible. The causes of abortion and of weak foals are many. In general, they may be classed as traumatic (due to an injury) and infectious.

The effects of certain active drugs, including some worm repellents, and the eating of some poisonous chemicals and plants and certain spoiled feeds may be mentioned as traumatic causes of abortion. Some types of illness, such as colic and parasitic infestation, may cause abortion. Mares may abort because of severe kicks or blows over the abdomen. Severe exertion and fatigue may endanger the life of the foal, while on the other hand lack of exercise may cause a weakening and break-down of the abdominal wall, with permanent injury to the mare. Light work each day until foaling time is to be recommended.

Bacterial infection is by far the greatest cause of abortions and stillbirths. Generalized infections such as influenza, infectious anemia, and similar febrile conditions may cause abortion. Infections that are localized in the reproductive tract, producing inflammation of the vagina, cervix, uterus, Fallopian tubes, and ovaries, may prevent conception or result in abortion. Infections of the reproductive tract of the male may be transmitted to the female and later cause abortion.

Infection by streptococci alone is said to cause 25 percent of all abortions. Abortions from this cause generally occur during early pregnancy. A large percentage of mares become infected at foaling time and do not overcome the infection before the first heat period, on or about the ninth day after foaling. A stallion may become infected when allowed to serve infected mares and may spread the infection to all the mares he serves. Streptococcic infection can be largely avoided through using non-infected mares and stallions and taking hygienic precautions. The vaginal examination prior to breeding is very essential, as previously mentioned. A bacterial culture should be made from any abnormal condition found at the examination following foaling. The culture is usually prepared from material obtained from the cervix. If the infection does not clear up by the first or second heat period, appropriate douches may be administered with benefit. It may be advisable to resort to the operation for partial closure of the vulva. Routine semen examinations of stallions should be made detect the presence of infection. It is essential to observe sanitary precautions, especially at foaling. Thorough disinfection of maternity stalls and the use of clean bedding will do much to prevent infection of clean animals.

An organism commonly causing joint ill in foals (*Shigella equirulis*) in some cases is passed from the dam to the fetus in the uterus. This infection is further discussed under Diseases of Newborn Foals.

The causative agent of contagious equine abortion is the organism known as *Salmonella abortivoequina*. Abortions due to this organism may occur at any stage of pregnancy, but usually from the fourth to the eighth month. Diagnosis may be made by examination of the blood for specific agglutinins. The disease may be largely controlled by the elimination of reacting mares and stallions as breeders and the vaccination of pregnant mares with a specific bacterin, especially in localities where abortion is prevalent. Aborting mares should be kept isolated. Discharges and all contaminated bedding, fetal membranes, and dead fetuses should be burned, and stalls should be thoroughly cleaned and disinfected. After a rest period, most mares will overcome the infection.

Large breeding establishments list many abortions under "unknown cause". In some studs as many as 50 percent or more of the mares may abort without showing any signs of illness, and bacterial cultures from the fetus and the mare may be negative. There are some indications that many such abortions may be due to a virus.

Dystocia and Retained Placenta

Dystocia (difficult labor) may result in the death of the foal and in extreme cases of the dam as well. While the entire process of labor normally requires a few hours, the actual expulsion of the foal should take place in less than half an hour. For mares requiring a longer time, the advice and assistance of a competent veterinarian should be immediately obtained. In some cases, traction applied to the fetus may be all that is required, but this is always a dangerous practice for one not trained in obstetrics as it may easily lead to the death of both dam and foal.

The placenta, or fetal membranes, commonly called the afterbirth, should come away in entirety from the mother within 2 hours after the birth of the foal. If any portion remains longer it is because of some abnormality which demands immediate professional attention. Delay in removal of all the placenta frequently results in septicemia (blood poisoning), laminitis (founder), or other serious complications.

Diseases of Newborn Foals

The death of newborn foals results not only in the loss of the stud fees, and of expected profit from the colts, but also in waste of the time and care devoted to the mares while in foal. Diseases of the newborn are due chiefly to infection; however, parasitism, faulty nutrition, and poor housing are important factors.

The diseases of foals caused by infection with micro-organisms include navel ill, joint in (lameness), pyosepticemia (blood poisoning), scours, and pneumonia. Almost any of the organisms causing these infections is capable of producing one or all of the symptoms.

The organisms that have most frequently been found to cause infections of the newborn are *Shigella equirulis* (syn. *Bacterium viscosum equi*), *Escherichia coli*, *Streptococcous*, and *Salmonella abortivoequina*. The last two are also common causes of abortion.

In *Shigella equirulis* infection the disease symptoms may appear at the time of or within 2 or 3 days after birth. There is a sudden onset with extreme prostration. The duration of symptoms is short, and death occurs early. During the course of the disease the pulse, temperature, and respiration are usually increased. Lameness may be pronounced in one or more joints, with visible enlargement. This organism is reported to cause a larger percentage of fatalities of young foals than any other one infection. Its habitat is believed to be in the digestive tract of the pregnant mare.

Symptoms of *Escherichia coli* infection are usually those of an acute septicemia, sometimes in association with inflammation of the joints and umbilicus (navel). Symptoms of infection usually appear at the time of birth or shortly thereafter, and as in the case of calves, in which it is a very serious problem, the mortality rate is high, death usually resulting in 1 to 4 days.

In streptococcic infection the disease usually appears 10 to 14 days after birth, causing lameness and swelling of joints followed by weakness and gradual loss of condition until death, the disease lasting 2 or 3 weeks. Some of the more chronic cases without general symptoms may recover. Streptococci have been found in a large percentage of unbred mares. These mares when bred are likely to abort or produce young that develop infection. This disease at the present time is thought to be one of the most important breeding diseases.

In paratyphoid (*Salmonella abortivoequina*) infection, the course of fatal cases of the disease is quite rapid, from 4 to 6 days, often accompanied by severe and persistent straining.

There is some difference of opinion among authorities as to the chief method of infection, whether it is prenatal (before birth) or postnatal (after birth); however, both types of infection should be considered important.

Prenatal, or intrauterine, infection of the foal takes place in the uterus (womb) of the dam before the foal is born. The infection may be present in the dam before she is bred, or it may be introduced by the stallion if he is infected or if he has previously bred other infected mares. Mechanical introduction of infection may result from unclean hands and equipment of operators, especially laymen who try to dilate the cervix (open up the mare for breeding) or diagnose pregnancy. If prenatal infection does not result in abortion and the mare carries the foal to the end of the gestation period, the colt is often born weak or develops navel ill within a few days and dies; if it does not die it becomes an unthrifty cripple that must be destroyed.

Postnatal infection primarily gains entrance to the body of the foal through the umbilicus after birth. This infection may be picked up from soil, bedding, or stables contaminated by other infected colts or mares that are discharging infective material.

The control of infectious diseases of the newborn foal by rigid sanitation and breeding hygiene is much more successful than treatment of an infected foal. Treatment is often nonspecific owing to the numerous different causes. Even when specific it often has very little therapeutic value owing to the rapid progress of the disease.

Control begins with hygiene before the mare is bred, as described in the previous section on Breeding Troubles.

After delivery, the nostrils of the foal should first be freed of membranes or obstruction of any kind; then the umbilical cord should be separated by traction if it has not separated naturally. This is accomplished by grasping the cord with both hands, pulling in such a manner as to separate it between the hands at a point 2 or 3 inches from the belly of the foal. The cord should not be ligated (tied), as this would prevent drainage. The umbilical stump should then be thoroughly saturated with a suitable disinfectant. Tincture of iodine is commonly used for this purpose. While one attendant holds the foal in a standing position, another holds a cupful of the solution up against its belly with the umbilical stump immersed in the fluid for about a minute. One application of the disinfectant in this manner is sufficient. The foal should be given a warm, nonirritating soap enema if it does not empty the contents of the lower bowel within the first 8 hours. This may be repeated as often as necessary until the normal yellow feces appear. Scours are not so common in foals as in calves. They may result from infection acquired from the udder and teats of the dam if these have become contaminated or from eating feces, straw, grass, and other foreign material or from overloading the stomach as a result of irregular nursing. Such irregularity may occur if the mare is taken away from the colt for a considerable length of time.

Treatment of infectious diseases of the foal, as previously stated, is usually unsuccessful because of the rapid progress of the disease, which does not allow sufficient time for diagnosis of the specific causative agent. Even when the specific cause is known, response to treatment is often unsatisfactory. However, with the first symptoms of sickness or lameness in the newborn foal, veterinary attention and advice are recommended. Blood transfusions from dam to foal have been given in all types of infection, with indications of favorable results.

In streptococcic infection, sulfanilamide has been reported to be of some value, and antistreptococcic serum and bacterins are sometimes used. The serum or bacterin should be specially prepared by a laboratory from the type of streptococcus concerned in the infection of the animals: since products prepared from other types of streptococcus may give no protection.

Except for administration of the dam's blood, treatment for *Shigella equirulis* infection has not proven to be very effective.

In *Escherichia coli* infection, antibacterial serum as used in calves for scours, the use of muzzles, and restriction of the diet may be of value.

Salmonella abortivoeqiona infection can be largely prevented by vaccinating the dam during the gestation period.

Lameness

Lameness frequently delays or even ends the training of show and race horses and commonly impedes farm work. It is, of course, not a disease but rather a manifestation of some structural or functional disorder of some part of the locomotive apparatus. On the other hand, a so-called false lameness is not uncommon in poorly conditioned or unwisely trained animals without any detectable abnormality.

The character and degree of lameness depend upon the nature and extent of the underlying ailments, which are many and varied. In, order to determine efficiently the origin of lameness, a thorough knowledge of anatomy and physiology is essential. In addition, it is helpful to recognize that every animal has a natural "way of going", which may or may not appear normal at first glance but which is compatible with the individual's constitution and conformation. Finally, a knowledge of pathology is necessary.

The duration of the lameness and whether it increases or decreases with continued exercise are points to be considered. If necessary the animal should be observed not only at rest but at all gaits if its condition permits. Enlargement or pain upon pressure or movement of any part is indicative of underlying disease. Sometimes X-rays assist in diagnosis. The nerves supplying certain portions of the leg are sometimes anesthetized, temporarily eliminating the sense of pain in the parts and permitting diagnosis through the process of elimination. The character of the lameness, that is, whether it involves support of weight or extension or flexion of the part, gives important clues as to the seat of the underlying trouble.

Causes

Lameness or impediments to the normal gait are observed in certain bone diseases, in azoturia, laminitis, lymphangitis, and miscellaneous wounds and diseases of the feet, which are discussed elsewhere in this article. There are numerous other causes. The diseases underlying lameness are chiefly inflammatory in nature. There are inflammations of bones, muscles, tendons, ligaments, joints, nerves, blood vessels, and skin, which may be the result of mechanical injury, infection, or both. Injuries develop either from accidental violence or from strains following forced training, overwork, improper shoeing, poorly fitted harness, and other largely preventable causes. Infection results chiefly from accidents. Some of the more common causes of lameness will be briefly discussed here.

Sprains

In an animal with good conformation and in good condition the muscles, tendons, and ligaments are marvelously coordinated in maintaining the bones in proper position, assisting in support of the body, and furnishing power for smooth movement. Sudden, severe, or prolonged exertion, especially in young or poorly conditioned animals, tends to cause undue strain in certain parts of the body and often produces stretching or laceration of the tissues, constituting what are commonly referred to as sprains. More severe injury may result in actual rupture of one or more of the major muscles, ligaments, or tendons, especially in the leg. In draft animals, sprains may result from the starting of heavy loads, long-continued, heavy hauling, or work where the footing is hard, rough, or slippery. Horses used in such sports as hunting, racing, and polo are frequently injured in this way as a result of over weighting, fast work on a wet track or field or in rough country, improperly balanced shoes, and the sudden stresses which are frequently encountered in competition. Injuries resulting from stumbling, falling, being kicked, or striking hurdles, mangers, etc., frequently occur. The conformation of some animals is faulty, and this, together with improper or incomplete conditioning before heavy work is imposed, may be a basic factor.

The initial injury is inevitably accompanied by more or less swelling and pain, depending on where the injury occurs. Injury of tendons or ligaments frequently involves some damage to the jointlike sheaths in which they are encased at points along their course, and even the periosteum (membranous covering of the bone) or the joints may become irritated. If the processes continue, the parts are apt to become infiltrated with fibrous tissue and even with calcium salts, leading to firm thickening, loss of elasticity, and contraction of the tissues. The continued irritation may lead to a great increase of the synovial fluid in the tendon sheaths or the joints. Sometimes bacteria, derived either from the outside or from some remote focus of infection within the body, invade the injured tissue.

If the initial, acute inflammatory changes do not recede and chronic infiltrations take place, such abnormalities as "bowed tendons," "bucked shins," hygroma (water knee), "calf knees," etc., result. The more extensive and chronic such changes are, the less is the likelihood of restoring the affected animal to complete soundness.

Foals are sometimes born with contracted tendons, as a result of which they are often unable to stand.

Arthritis

Arthritis is an inflammation of an articulation, or joint, between two or more bones. It occurs primarily or secondarily as a result of injury, involving other factors such as conformation, and may or may not be complicated by bacterial invasion. When foreign objects perforate the joint capsule, infection invariably follows. The result is extreme lameness, accompanied by fever and other constitutional disturbances. Chronic arthritis results in enlargement and impaired movement of the joint.

Luxations (Dislocations)

The displacement of bones from their normal coordinated position constitutes a luxation. The patella (kneecap in man), located in the stifle joint, is sometimes displaced upward or outward and either an extreme straightening of the hind leg in a forward position or a relaxed state in which it will not support the body weight results. Such animals are said to be "stifled." Other less frequent luxations occur in the shoulder, knee fetlock, and hip joints.

Luxation, particularly of the patella, sometimes occurs after debilitating diseases such as influenza and pneumonia. It is encountered in colts with joint in or rickets, or may result from injury, and in some cases it appears as a congenital defect. Serious injury is the usual cause in the case of joints other than the stifle.

Affections of the Nerves and Blood Vessels

The nerves of the legs are generally fairly well protected from injury by other tissues, but injuries do occasionally occur that result in more or less severe lameness. These lamenesses are to be distinguished from defects in the gait attributable to damage in the central nervous system (brain and spinal cord) such as develops in encephalomyelitis and other diseases. Injury of the suprascapular nerve results in a bulging of the shoulder and may be the cause of muscular atrophy or wasting, which is commonly known as sweeny, or swinney. In some bases of difficult foaling the obturator nerve on either or both sides may be compressed between the dam's pelvis and some part of the fetus. As a result, the muscles holding the legs in toward the body may be paralyzed and a spreading of one or both legs occurs. Paralysis of the foreleg may follow injury of the brachial or radial nerves. Minor injury leads to awkward use of the leg, while severe injury results in complete limpness of the entire leg. Tumors may press upon the nerves controlling certain muscles, causing symptoms of paralysis.

Normal tone and function of the body muscles is primarily dependent upon the supply of blood they receive. Inflammation of the blood vessels, chiefly the arteries, may occur in the legs as well as other parts of the body as the result of invasion by blood strongyles, or palisade worms. The walls become thickened, and clots form in the iliac, femoral, and other arteries of the leg. Injury may lead to the formation of similar lesions. In consequence, the blood supply to the legs is more or less decreased. Thrombosis, or clot formation, in the iliac artery produces a characteristic type of lameness with which there may be profuse sweating, trembling, widely dilated nostrils, and rapid breathing. The attack may disappear as rapidly as it developed, leaving the animal entirely normal to all appearances, or apart of the clot may be dislodged into the blood stream and become fixed in a vessel in some vital organ, such as the brain, which may cause death. The attacks of lameness somewhat resemble azoturia in appearance, but in this case they may recur at any time, whereas in azoturia there is no relapse.

Fractures and Stringhalt

Fractures or broken bones may result from severe injury or extreme strain. The symptoms are dependent upon the location and extent of the damage. The affected animal does not always collapse as a result of the break but nearly always reveals extreme pain when compelled to move. Disturbance of normal alinement and relationship between the bones, crepitation, or grating sounds, when the leg is manipulated, and X-ray findings are elements of diagnosis. Most fractures of the leg bones of horses or mules are not amenable to treatment under ordinary conditions, but in the case of some valuable animals, especially if they are young and tractable, it is practical for the veterinarian to attempt treatment. Unusually ideal conditions, however, are always required.

Stringhalt consists in spasmodic contractions of the muscles of the hind leg as a result of which the foot is pulled or jerked upward. The ailment usually develops slowly, progressively increasing in severity, but it rarely leads to complete loss of service ability. Most often it affects only one leg, though both hind legs may be involved. The symptoms are likely to be most marked when the affected animal is first taken from the stall or when it is backed. In some cases the flexion of the leg is so sudden and violent that the animal falls to the ground. With continued exercise, the condition tends to improve, finally disappearing after a short time in most cases, only to reassert itself after a period of rest. By some it is considered a form of neurosis; others believe it to be hereditary, and still other theories have been advanced. No known line of treatment is successful in all calies. Various neurectomies (severing of nerves) and tenotomies (severing" of tendons) are performed, often with apparent benefit. Medicinal treatment is not known to be of any avail.

Prevention and Treatment of Lameness

With good husbandry, including prevention of wounds and wise care of the feet, there is little lameness in horses or mules of sound constitution, free from hereditary defects or seriously inferior conformation. Patience and understanding should always be practiced in training animals. All parts of the harness should be adjusted properly. Measures taken to modify a horse's gait should be developed gradually. These precautions will limit unnecessary strains which might lead to ailments causing lameness. Immediate attention should be given to the slightest indication of lameness. Delay or unwise treatment may lead to needless complications or incurable conditions.

The first principle of the treatment of a lame animal is rest. The second is accurate diagnosis. Third, it should be understood that no one drug, combination of drugs, or system of treatment is applicable to all cases, even of the same one of the many aliments which result in lameness. Rest alone may be all that is required to correct some simple abnormalities. If the nature and site of the trouble have been determined, cold packs may be applied to the part. Again, alternate hot and cold packs or repeated soaking of the part in a saturated solution of Epsom salts may be advisable. Elastic or other bandages are sometimes applied to sprains with benefit. Various astringent lotions are sometimes used.

Irritants or blistering substances applied in the early stages of most lamenesses are harmful. Only when the condition responsible for the lameness fails to respond to rest and conservative treatment or when chronic changes are present should counter irritation be used. It may be advisedly employed to produce a superficial inflammation in the case of chronic lesions of a tendon, tendon sheath, joint, or bone. Cautery, or "firing," may be used either with or without the adjunct of a so-called blistering agent.

Firing is an accepted form of treatment for chronic ailments that do not yield to conservative treatment and rest. It should not be used, indiscriminately by the untrained and cannot be expected to result in the complete disappearance of chronic proliferations (abnormal growth) of tissue, including bone. The Irons used in this process are of various shapes for different purposes and are heated by electricity, chemicals, or fire. Care and Judgment are necessary to be sure that sufficient but not excessive counter irritation results. A blistering ointment is often used following firing. After such treatment it is best to tie up the animal for a few days or until the acute inflammation subsides, after which it is a common practice to remove the shoes, trim the feet, and the put the animal on pasture for a time.

Wounds causing lameness are treated according to their extent and location, with due regard for the control of infection and the preservation or restoration of normal function in the affected part.

Enlargements of joints or tendon sheaths due to an accumulation of fluid are usually treated by withdrawing the fluid under sterile conditions; this in some cases is followed by injection of antiseptic solution and counter irritation or bandaging.

Special manipulations are required to reduce a luxation. This is usually relatively easy to accomplish, but the condition is apt to recur in many cases if the injury is severe or if treatment has been delayed.

Contracted tendons, especially in foals, frequently require surgical attention and the temporary use of specially made supports.

Advanced cases of sweeny in which marked shrinking of the muscle has taken place are commonly treated by injection with various forms of iodine in solution or other substances to stimulate the formation of new tissue.

Some fractures of certain bones, if detected immediately after the injury takes place and if not too great damage has resulted, will heal under competent care. In most cases, however, humane destruction of the animal is advised by the attending veterinarian on practical grounds.

Bone Diseases

Probably diseases of the bones are responsible for more lay-offs of draft horses and mules than any other one class of ailments. The services of large numbers of racing and other sporting horses are temporarily and in some cases permanently lost through the same cause.

The chief feature of most bone diseases of solipeds is exostosis, or abnormal growth of bone. This arises primarily from faulty feeding which provides an insufficiency of the minerals necessary for the production and preservation of normal bone. Accessory factors are strains and other injuries such as are discussed under the heading Lameness. Animals with defective conformation are particularly apt to develop these conditions. Improper shoeing may be a contributing cause. Finally, heredity is believed to influence the occurrence of at least some bone diseases. Spavin and ringbone are among the diseases that disqualify a stallion or jack for registration for public service, except as an unsound animal, in many States. Unusually, nervous animal, even without defects in conformation or ancestry, appear to be subject to spavin.

The spavin considered here is that involving the bones of the tarsus, or hock, rather than so-called bog spavin, which consists of an accumulation of synovial fluid in and around the joint. Bone spavin usually develops gradually. At first the lameness disappears after the animal goes a short distance, only to return after a rest. "Warming out" becomes less frequent as the disease advances, and there are large bony enlargements (exostosis) of the joints. To the experienced observer, the character of the lameness is quite distinctive even in the absence of definite enlargement. The exostosis, which is usually, greatest on the inside of the joint, is most easily detected by viewing the hock from between the forelegs, at an angle from near the shoulder, or from behind. The condition is especially prevalent in animals with small, weak hocks.

Ringbone is an exostosis involving the first and second phalangeal bones, that is, those immediately below the fetlock. Animals with short, upright pasterns seem to be especially predisposed to this condition. It is classified as high, low, and in other ways, according to its location and extent. The lameness of ringbone is especially manifested when the affected animal is required to step from side to side. Marked flinching then occurs when weight is borne on the affected leg, even though no lameness may be revealed when the animal goes in a straight line. The lameness is frequently irregular at first, often being overlooked entirely by the driver or rider, but it finally becomes more or less constant and is attended by plainly visible bony enlargement of the pastern.

Sidebones consist of ossification, or formation of bone, in the lateral cartilages, which are attached to the third phalangeal bone within the hoof, extending above the hoof at the coronet (point of junction of skin and hoof). These cartilages, one on each side of each foot, are normally very resilient, forming a shock-absorbing apparatus within the hoof and presumably assisting in the circulation of blood in the foot. The ossification of these structures greatly disturbs the normal elasticity of the internal part of the foot and the changes in its shape which occur under the influence of the weight of the body, The hardening of the cartilages due to the formation of bone has the effect of cramping the structures of the internal part of the foot, and lameness is inevitable. Sidebones are especially frequent in heavy draft types of horses. They occur chiefly in the front feet.

Splints are not, as some laymen believe, due to growth of a great mass of new bone on the cannon, or shank, bone. The condition consists rather of a comparatively limited exostosis between the cannon bone (large metacarpal) and the small splint bones (small metacarpals), which are situated one on each side of the rear surface of the cannon bone, just below the knee. The splint bones are attached to the cannon by ligaments, forming apart of the carpus, or knee, joint at their upper extremity. The trouble begins with inflammation due to strain or injury of the periosteum or the ligamentous attachment between the cannon and split bones. The condition is quite common during the training of young animals, rarely being encountered in those over 6 to 8 years of age.

The animal may walk normally but is very lame at the trot, nodding the head with each step. The bony enlargements which appear some time after lameness begins usually occur on the inside splint bones. They may be the size of a pea or as large as a small marble. Before the proliferation of bone occurs, the parts are sensitive to pressure. When, as sometimes happens, the condition develops in both forelegs, the lameness is not readily detectable.

The term "navicular" is used indiscriminately to designate various diseases affecting the structures which form the coffin joint–that between the second and third phalanges within the hoof. More strictly speaking, navicular disease refers to inflammations involving the navicular bone (third sesamoid), the deep flexor tendon, and the bursa podotrochlearis, or navicular bursa. Usually the disease occurs in one forefoot, though sometimes both are affected. Only occasionally does it develop in the hind feet. Lameness is the first indication. The animal is inclined to stumble, and there is a stilted gait due to shortening of the stride. In advanced cases involving only one foot, there is a characteristic "pointing"–advancing the affected foot well in front of its mate when standing.

The general group of bone diseases classed as rickets (rachitis) and bighead (osteoporosis, osteomalacia, and osteitis fibrosa) are discussed in some detail in the article on Nutritional Diseases of Farm Animals.

Prevention and Treatment of Bone Diseases

Proper feeding is essential for the development of sound bones in horses and mules as well as other animals. It should begin with the dam and is of great importance for the foal and the developing animal.

Horse breeders desirous of producing sound animals should have a thorough understanding of good conformation. For example, in breeding stock, pasterns that are exceptionally long and sloping or too short and upright are to be especially avoided. Small, weak hocks, poorly alined legs, and poor feet also are important contributing factors in lameness, particularly that attributable to bone diseases.

There is considerable evidence that certain bone ailments, notably spavin and ringbone, are especially prevalent in the offspring of certain animals. There is the suggestion of such a hereditary influence in other diseases of the bones. This is reflected in faulty conformation or constitutional weakness.

Care and judgment in the management of horses and mules, including their shoeing, can assist in lessening strains and injuries which may lead directly or indirectly to the disabling bone diseases.

The principles of treatment of bone diseases are outlined under the heading Prevention and Treatment of Lameness. It should be realized, however, that long-continued diseases of the bone frequently result in irreparable damage. Thus, both spavin and ringbone commonly lead, to ankylosis, or complete fusion of the bones of apart or all the Involved joint. If the processes of the disease cannot be arrested early by rest and appropriate treatment, permanent damage must be expected to follow. In this event, serviceability rather than soundness is the goal of treatment. Specially designed shoes are frequently prescribed for such cases, in conjunction with changing of the proportions or angles of the hoof by appropriate trimming.

Foot Ailments

"No foot, no horse" concisely expresses a principle well understood by experienced horsemen. The horse or mule without sound feet is so apt to be incapacitated, either temporarily or permanently, that every precaution possible should be taken. A number of troubles attributable directly or indirectly to improper management or to faulty conformation are briefly discussed here. More or less lameness develops sooner or later as a result of any of these conditions.

As a preliminary, it may be well to consider the normal foot of the horse. The hoof of solipeds may well be compared with the human toenail except that it completely encases the digit. The hoof consists of a more or less dense, fibrous, horny material derived from the skin at the coronet (the spongy, padlike tissue just above the hoof at its junction with the skin).Within this case of horn are bones, tendons, ligaments, nerves, and an intricate network of blood vessels. The hoof wall and sole are attached to the underlying structures by means of so-called sensitive and insensitive laminae. These consist of minute leaf like structures which are closely united in dovetailed fashion. Unyielding as the hoof appears to be, it has been proved that it expands and contracts in synchronized waves when the animal moves on it, particularly at the heels and the coronary cushion. Even the sole of the loot, which is superimposed over a pad like structure known as the plantar cushion, flattens out when weight is borne. The so-called lateral cartilages (described in connection with sidebones,) are an important part of this normal expansion and contraction.

The nutriment for the structures of the foot is received from the blood, the flow of which is largely controlled by the expansion and contraction of the parts described. The hoof wall grows at the rate of about one-fourth of an inch a month, being pushed down from the coronet regularly all around the foot. Growth is favored by moisture and good nutrition and general health as well as by exercise. The unshod hoof grows more rapidly than one with shoes.

The white line at the junction of the wall with the sole marks the point of union between the minute horny leaves of the sole and those of the wall. In shoeing, the nails are driven through the hoof at a point just outside this line. The sole is marked by a deep, V-shaped cleft, outlined on each side by the bars, which are a continuation of the wall. The pyramidal or triangle-shaped horny structure within the lines of the V formed by the bars is known as the frog. The entire sole of the hoof, as well as the walls, covers highly sensitive-tissue richly supplied with nerves and blood vessels.

By conformation is meant the general form, outline, and arrangement of parts. The conformation of the ideal foot varies somewhat with the type of animal and even with the breed. Generally speaking, the well-shaped hoof is roughly like a cone from above downward. The print made by the hoof is generally oval, being slightly greater in length than in width. The walls of the hoof slope gradually and evenly outward from above and are free from deep grooves or bulges. The substance of the normal hoof is dense and firm but not brittle, and it has a distinctive gloss, the result of a varnish like substance called periople, which lessens the evaporation of the water normally present in the horn. The bars are well defined, strong, and widely spaced. There is no compressed narrowing of the foot at the heel, and the frog is clean and well-formed.

The feet should be centered on a perpendicular line from the point of the buttocks through the hock and fetlock in the hind leg and from the shoulder through the knee and fetlock in the front leg. Viewed from the side, the axis through the fetlock, pastern, and hoof should consist of a straight, unbroken line forming an angle of about 34° with the base of the foot. The hoof at the heel should generally be approximately one-third as long as in front.

The foot of the mule or ass is considerably smaller and rounder than the foot of the horse. In addition, the pastern is generally more erect, giving the hoof a comparatively "stumpy" appearance.

Brittle Hoofs, Spongy Hoofs, Crooked Foot, and Contracted Foot

As the term "brittle hoofs" indicates, there may develop an abnormally dry state of the horn. The hoof becomes almost of the consistency of stone and chips and cracks easily. Brittle hoofs tend to encourage contracted heels and lead to difficulties in shoeing. It has been observed that short, cobby animals of certain breeds commonly have this defect. Long-continued dryness or stabling on dry, hard floors is conducive to the trouble. Repeated applications of certain hoof dressings on show animals may be a contributing cause. In cases of brittle hoofs, it is often advisable to remove the shoes, trim the feet, and reshoe, under a veterinarian's supervision whenever possible. The bearing surface should be made as level as possible, and thin nails should be used, placed in the strongest parts of the hoof wall. When a level bearing cannot be established, a hoof cement; is sometimes used advantageously. A hoof ointment containing such substances as turpentine, tar, and wax in an oily or fatty base is often beneficial.

The opposite of brittle hoofs, spongy hoofs are characterized by abnormally soft, nonresistant horn. This condition is a common characteristic of certain breeds and is encountered in animals kept on marshy ground and those of a so-called lymphatic type. Such feet are predisposed to canker and corns. Special care must be taken in shoeing spongy or soft hoofs. Excessive paring of the sole and hot fitting of the shoe are special hazards. Animals with such hoofs are prone to develop dry horn and contracted feet unless particular care is taken.

The term "crooked foot" denotes a foot with one side wall higher than the other. Sometimes the hoof wall is curved in or out on one or both sides. This is often attributable to inherited faulty conformation with "toeing in" or "toeing out," but it may be brought about by unequal paring of the foot or by bad shoeing. Gradual lowering of the high side of a crooked foot by repeated trimming will tend to improve the condition, but complete and permanent correction is impossible when the trouble results from faulty conformation of the leg. Special shoes are sometimes applicable, but they should be frequently reset.

Flat feet with low, weak heels, Improperly shod feet in which the frog does not receive normal ground pressure, and feet excessively dried out during a long period of dry, hot weather are apt to become contracted, chiefly at the heels. Excessive paring of the bars may also be a factor. Contraction of long standing is obstinate and impractical to treat in many cases. Animals with such feet are often much better off without shoes. Going thus barefooted permits natural pressure on the frog, and spreading of the heels is the natural result. In shoeing, the bars and frog should be let alone as much as possible, and expansion or other special shoes may be applied. Hoof ointments assist in softening the horn, which tends to become hard.

Sand Crack, Corns and Thrush

Cracks or splits in the hoof wall following the direction of the horn fibers are classified according to their position as toe crack, quarter crack, or sand crack of the frog or sole. Sand crack is attributable fundamentally to faulty conformation, being found also in animals with brittle hoofs. Rasping of the periople from the outer surface of the hoof wall tends to weaken the wall, promoting sand cracks. They sometimes arise also from purely accidental causes in wholly normal hoofs. They are not particularly serious if the underlying sensitive structures are not involved. Unfortunately, the veterinarian is seldom consulted until the injury is deep-seated and lameness is apparent, and treatment is then not always wholly satisfactory.

Sand cracks are treated according to their location and extent. In simple cases, blistering the coronet with an irritating substance will sometimes sufficiently stimulate horn growth to overcome the crack. The margins of the crack may be drawn together by a skilled horseshoer and clamped with a well-placed horseshoe nail or clamps especially designed for the purpose. Special shoeing is sometimes advantageously employed. Grooves may be cut around the crack to immobilize the hoof wall, thus permitting healing. Finally, in complicated cases, the portion of horn involved in the crack may be removed by cutting or burning, but frequent dressing and a protracted rest are necessary until new horn fills the uncovered space.

The term "corn" to the veterinarian indicates the changes that follow the bruising of the sensitive sole of the hoof, usually between the bar and the wall. The injury is more common in the forefeet and on the inner side. The bruise is accompanied by hemorrhage and consequent discoloration from red to brown, greenish, or yellow. There is pain in the swollen structures. A dry corn is one fortunately unattended by excessive inflammatory changes. A considerable amount of inflammatory exudate, or discharge, is present in a moist corn, and pus is found in the suppurating corn.

Corns are considered by most authorities as basically attributable to faults in conformation (wide, flat. feet with low heels; high, contracted heels; long or overgrown hoofs). Direct injury in connection with excessive moisture or dryness and stable filth and excessive paring of the sole, bars, or frog by overzealous farriers are also contributing causes.

Treatment of corns is not always satisfactory, especially in cases of very long standing. Paring of the sole is not always advisable but may be necessary for the liberation of pus. When shoes are applied, one of the main objectives is provision of frog pressure. So-called bar shoes are put on after careful leveling of the foot, Suppurating corns may require frequent special dressings.

A degenerative condition of the frog characterized by a black, offensive pus is called thrush. Often the first indication of the trouble to the casual observer is the characteristic stench. Thrush is caused by an infection first of the horn and later of the sensitive structures. The horn is normally resistant to bacterial invasion but may become deteriorated through long-continued exposure to excessively wet or filthy stalls or paddocks or extended exposure to extremely dry footing, especially in cases of contracted feet. Thrush is more common in the hind feet. Lameness nearly always attends it sooner or later. It is necessary first to trim away all the diseased horn, exposing the depths of the process for antiseptic treatment. The foot should be so trimmed or shod as to restore and preserve normal frog pressure.

Canker, Grease Heel, and Quittor

Symptoms of canker are seldom noticed early, as the disease progresses slowly and practically without pain at first. An inflammatory change in the horn-forming tissue causes secretion of a serous fluid instead of the normally produced horny cells. Eventually the frog and even part of the sole may be separated from the underlying sensitive tissue. Instead of normal horn being formed, there is often a fungoid mass. Deep in the tissue surrounding the lesson there is frequently an accumulation of fetid, cheeselike material. As a result of fungoid growth, the horny sole and frog, and sometimes the entire foot, become deformed.

The disease is confused with thrush and by some is considered as an advanced form of that disease. The exact cause remains undetermined. Certain factors, however, appear to be conducive to canker. Continued standing in dampness and filth or any condition which removes the natural counter pressure on the frog may be suspected as a predisposing cause of this disease as well as of thrush.

Canker is a difficult condition to treat in advanced cases. Surgical removal of the abnormal growth followed by application of a hot iron, packing with an antiseptic pad, and shoeing with specially designed canker-dressing shoes are the essentials of the usual procedure.

"Grease heel" is a term commonly applied to an inflammation of the skin of the pastern and fetlock. The specific cause is unknown, but it is usually seen in heavy horses with coarse, thick legs when such horses are kept in damp, insanitary stables or are long subjected to mud and filth without proper cleaning.

At first there are swelling, and redness of the skin, with some itching. Later there is an increased secretion from the sebaceous glands in the affected region, over which the hair stands erect, glued together by the oily secretion, which has an offensive odor. The skin, at first moist and painful, tends to become thickened, and finally, after several months, fungoid masses commonly referred to as "grapes" may be formed. The hind legs are more commonly affected.

In treating grease heel it is advisable first to clip closely all hair of the affected areas. The region should when be thoroughly cleaned with mild soap and water. Following this, various astringent, antiseptic substances are applied at regular intervals. In cases of long standing in which wartlike growths are present these must be removed surgically and the wounds suitably dressed until healing takes place.

The opening at the coronet of one or more sinuses, or pus-discharging passages, is called quittor. The pus originates primarily from a necrotic (dead) lateral cartilage; later, any of the internal structures of the foot may be involved.

Infection may gain entrance through calk wounds,. inflammatory conditions of the skin over the coronet, a suppurating corn, a puncture wound in the foot, sand cracks, etc. Cartilage is poorly nourished by the blood; when once it is injured and infected, necrosis invariably follows.

There is usually more or less severe inflammatory swelling around the opening, which is painful. Pus of a grayish color, often streaked with blood, is discharged almost constantly. In chronic cases, hoof deformities result from the disturbed circulation in the coronary band. The deeper the sinus and the more copious the discharge, the poorer the chances of recovery.

Treatment depends upon the degree and extent of the damage. In a few cases, simple drainage and antiseptic treatment result favorably. In most, however, a radical surgical operation involving the removal of all diseased tissue becomes necessary. Frequent dressing is required, and the convalescent period may be quite prolonged.

Prevention of Foot Ailments

From the foregoing, it will be seen that most of the foot abnormalities arise either from inherited poor conformation or improper care of the feet. Poor conformation can be largely avoided by proper selection of animals, either for breeding or for work. The inexperienced should not hesitate to consult a veterinarian in this connection. The application of shoes is an unnatural necessity for many, if not most, horses and mules. If improperly done, injury inevitably follows.

Here are some do's and don'ts in taking proper care of the feet of horses and mules:

The feet of stabled animals should be trimmed, removing all excess growth of the hoof wall, at least once a month. Pastured animals should receive this attention at least every 2 months.

Shoes should be reset or replaced every month. Failure to change, the shoes results in the natural growth of the hoof carrying the heel too far beneath the foot for proper bearing.

The feet should be thoroughly cleaned with a blunt stick and sponge or brush and water after every day's work. It is considered a bad practice to use the currycomb below the knees or hocks. A brush or cloth is preferable.

The pasterns and fetlocks should receive special attention in grooming each day, particularly after work in mud or snow.

Stalls should be roomy, clean, well-bedded, and well-drained. During protracted dry weather, the hoofs are apt to become excessively dry, especially if the animals stand on concrete or brick floors. If floors are of dirt, considerable care should be taken to keep them smooth and well-graded. If the hoofs show signs of dryness, periodic soaking for an hour or more at a time in clean water is advantageous.

When an animal is shod, rasping the outer wall and cutting the bars, sole, or frog should not be permitted except under a veterinarian's supervision.

Shoes of other than conventional design should not be applied except under the direction of a veterinarian.[3]

Skin Diseases

Afflictions of the skin are relatively infrequent in horses and mules except under improper management, which contributes greatly to the occurrence and spread of such diseases, both infectious and noninfectious.

The skin is an integral part of the body as a whole, and, as such, it reflects either general health or abnormality. Thus, excessive sweating (hyperhidrosis) occurs in certain febrile diseases, failure to sweat (anhidrosis) may be an indication of general debility from various causes, and itching (pruritis) may be traceable to dietary excesses or deficiencies. Hematidrosis, or so-called sweating of blood, is not due to the actual secretion of blood by the sweat glands but rather to mixing of blood with the sweat as a result of a general circulatory disease, as in purpura hemorrhagica. Rational feeding and moderate exercise or work, together with general stable hygiene, promote the health of the skin as well as that of the rest of the body, and when diseases of the skin occur under these conditions they are generally attributable to inflammation caused externally by parasites or irritating chemical. substances.

Itching may occur in animals as a result of chronic bowel irritation, chronic kidney disease, failure to shed or delay in shedding the coat, or the long-continued feeding of a restricted diet. It is present in some cases of alopecia (falling of the hair) and ringworm, and it is an almost constant symptom in eczema, pediculosis (lousiness), and mange. Intense itching frequently occurs in animals developing rabies.

Erythema of the skin, or redness due to congestion of blood, is a result of excessive or exclusive feeding of certain feeds such as

---

3 The elements of conformation and shoeing are discussed in Farmers' Bulletins 779, How: to Select a Sound Horse, and 1535, Farm Horseshoeing.

clovers, potatoes, and distillers' grains, and in some cases it occurs in animals on an exclusive ration of alfalfa. It may developed during the course of administration of certain drugs, from friction, or from excessive heat, cold, or sunshine. It is seen in eczema and parasitic infestations and in the course of various infectious diseases.

Dandruff, an accumulation of branlike scales on the skin, is observed in eczema, mange, iodine poisoning, louse infestations., and some cases of chronic digestive diseases.

The diagnosis of skin diseases, which is generally essential before satisfactory treatment can be applied, is often very difficult for even the most experienced veterinarian. There are, however, certain more or less common skin diseases with which the horseman should become at least superficially acquainted in order that he may, as far as possible, avoid them and realize the difficulties to be encountered in diagnosis and treatment. A brief discussion of these follows.

Eczema, Acne, and Urticaria (Hives)

Eczema is defined as a superficial, or surface, inflammation of the skin and is classified for descriptive purposes into several types not of special interest in this discussion. It is most common in the spring, especially in old horses, in which it is often chronic. Vesicles (small water blisters), papules (pimples), or dandruff are common indications of the disease. An eruption with more or less severe itching appears over the body generally or on any part of it. When confined to certain areas, it frequently appears first at the base of the tail or mane.

The vesicles rupture, discharging their contents and matting the hair. Rubbing the parts leads to loss of hair and rawness of the skin. Later, crusts or dandruff appear. During the course of the disease, bacterial infection may take place, and deep infiltration by pus sometimes develops. Eczema sometimes affects several horses at a time in the same stable as if it were contagious. It is aggravated by the use of irritating soaps or solutions. Sometimes it appears so much like mange that differentiation can be made only by failure to find mites. The condition tends to improve during cool or cold weather, becoming worse during warm periods.

The causes of eczema are not exactly known, but they are considered to be variable. Accumulations of mud and snow in the coat, insanitary stables, and lack of grooming to remove accumulation of dirt and sweat appear to be accessory factors. Underlying. causes may be a basic sensitiveness to certain feeds or chronic digestive disturbances.

Acne is sometimes called summer mange, although it is not actually mange. It consists of an inflammation of the hair follicles and sebaceous glands caused by pus-forming bacteria. The lesions of the disease, which are either small pimples or larger boillike formations, may occur on any part of the body but are more commonly found in parts rubbed by the harness or saddle. The bacteria appear thus to be rubbed into the pores and follicles.

Urticaria is a manifestation of anaphylaxis (an intoxication due to introduction of a substance, usually a protein, to which the animal is sensitive). It is characterized by the sudden appearance of numbers of rounded, elevated areas in the skin over the head and neck or on the body. The circumscribed swellings are attributable to the infiltration of the skin by edema. The condition sometimes appears in several infectious diseases, and in purpura hemorrhagica; as a result of contact with irritants, such as plants of the genus *Urtica* (stinging nettles) or irritating chemicals; following insect bites; as an anaphylactic reaction to certain feeds; or as a result of absorption of toxic substances from the gastrointestinal tract.

Light Sensitization, Ringworm, and Lymphangitis

Light sensitization is manifested almost exclusively in white-skinned or spotted animals. In the latter, only the white areas are involved. It apparently is induced by the consumption of certain plants, chiefly legumes, the pigments of which under certain conditions form a substance in the blood that sensitizes the body cells to sunlight, resulting in edematous; or watery infiltrations of the skin and underlying tissues. Inflammation of the membranes of the mouth, colic, jaundice, and even symptoms of brain disturbances may also occur.

Following edema of the skin with or without the formation of vesicles, the skin surface becomes dry and encrusted. Itching may be occur. Gangrene of the skin (death of the tissue) may result, leading to the sloughing of the tissue and leaving a raw surface which may be attacked by pus-forming bacteria.

The plants most commonly implicated in this trouble, which may affect cattle and other animals as well as horses, include Swedish clover (*Trifolium hybridum*), red clover (*Trifolium pratense*), vetch (*Vicia sativa*), and St. Johnswort (*Hypericum* species).

The remedy is to change the pasture or hay and keep the animals out of the sunshine for a time. In severe cases, mild protective dressings are sometimes applied to the most seriously affected areas of the skin.

Ringworm is a contagious disease caused by certain microscopic molds (*Trichophyta, Mierospora*, etc.). The disease may be transmitted to man and other animals.

Rounded, scaly patches with sparse hair occur on the skin of any part of the body, but chiefly the shoulder, breast, flank, croup, back, or head and neck, and less often on the legs or the abdomen. Asbestos like crusts may be formed, and the skin generally has a grayish or yellowish powdery or warty appearance in the affected regions. After a time the originally affected areas tend to return to normal, the hair grows in and the skin become soft and smooth. But new patches appear in adjacent areas, eventually spreading over most of the body. Ringworm in horses usually causes little itching.

The organism responsible for the condition is usually readily demonstrable microscopically, and it can be cultivated in the laboratory from the scales and hairs from the affected skin. Strict sanitation is an essential in the control of ringworm.

In the nutrition of the body the blood itself does not come in direct contact with the tissue cells. The cells are directly nourished through the medium of a fluid known as lymph, which is derived from the blood. Lymph circulates about the body through channels known as lymph vessels. Lymphangitis is an inflammation of these vessels.

Strictly speaking, this condition is not, of course, a disease of the skin, but since its outward manifestations involve the skin, it is included here. There are at least three main forms which affect solipeds–sporadic lymphangitis ("big-leg" or "weed"), ulcerative lymphangitis, and mycotic or epizootic lymphangitis.

Sporadic lymphangitis occurs chiefly in heavy-legged animals which have been held in the stall on full feed for a number of days between periods of work. For this reason; it is sometimes referred to as Monday-morning disease, as is azoturia also. It appears that the lack of usual exercise and continuation of a full ration, especially it highly nitrogenous one, results in slowing the flow of lymph, which in turn leads to a "filling" or "stocking" of one or more of the legs, chiefly the hind legs. Poorly groomed animals with dirty legs or those with cracked heels, thrush, and similar ailments are especially prone to the condition, and it is assumed that the lesions harboring various pus-forming organisms lead to infection of the lymph stream and consequently the vessels. In acute cases there may be fever, chills, and extreme lameness. Drops of yellowish, glairy liquid, resembling white of egg, may accumulate on the leg. This acute stage may last 2 or 3 days, with gradual improvement, or it may persist and lead to a chronic affection. Some animals appear to recover only to develop the same condition later. Chronic cases develop a permanent thickening of the skin known as elephantiasis.

Ulcerative lymphangitis is attributed to infection by germs known as corynebacteria. In this disease, infection apparently takes place through wounds, chiefly in the feet, the lesions usually being confined to the hind legs, beginning above the fetlocks. In addition to a doughy swelling of the leg, small abscesses develop along the course of the lymph vessels and burst, discharging a yellow or blood-stained pus. The resulting raw ulcers tend to heal in a few weeks, leaving hairless scars. Succeeding crops of abscesses and ulcers appear, and the lymph glands become involved. Even the internal organs may be affected. The causative germ can be cultivated in the laboratory.

Mycotic lymphangitis is attributed to a yeast like fungus known as *Cryptococcus farciminosus* Rivolta. Infection is believed to take place through wounds on any part of the body, chiefly the legs. The lymph vessels adjacent to the wound become prominent, and nodules varying from the size of a pea to that of a walnut develop along their course. These burst, discharging a thick white or fainty yellow pus, and red ulcers with little tendency to heal are formed. The organism causing the disease can be grown in artificial media.

All of these forms of lymphangitis may resemble glanders, and tests for that disease as well as laboratory examinations may be required for the exact diagnosis.

Treatment and Prevention

Accurate diagnosis is an especially important first step in the treatment of diseases of the skin. From the standpoint of symptoms, many of these ailments are identical in the eyes of the layman, while to the veterinarian clear points of differentiation may be readily apparent. However, very close study and laboratory examination are frequently desirable.

Just as any animal suspected of having an infectious disease should be isolated, so should those with any indication of communicable skin diseases. Even though the veterinarian may later determine that the disease is not transmissible to other animals, better care of the affected animal frequently results from its separation from others in the stable.

Because there are few specific remedies for skin diseases and these are not necessarily applicable in all cases of a given affection, no detailed discussion of medical treatment will be attempted here. Suffice it to say that such a preparation as tincture of iodine is not applicable in every case of ringworm, nor is an acceptable mange remedy necessarily effective in the treatment of eczema; in fact, it is more apt to be harmful.

Clean stables and regular grooming are of the greatest importance in promoting general health and preventing and treating diseases of the skill. Regular cleaning of harness saddles, blankets, grooming equipment, etc., are parts of good husbandry. If communicable skill diseases appear in the stable, disinfection of the equipment becomes necessary.

Noninfectious and nonparasitic skin diseases are often aggravated if not directly caused by poor condition, which can frequently be improved by modifications or complete changes in the diet. Animals not being regularly worked should have some exercise every day, if, possible and the quantity of their ration should be regulated according to the activity.

Prescription and application of medicinal agents should be left to the attending veterinarian.

Abnormalities of the Teeth

Deciduous, or milk, teeth, 24 in number, appear in the horse's mouth early in life and are much smaller than the second or permanent set, which number 36 in the mare and 42 in the male horse.[4] The majority of these erupt or replace the deciduous set at 2½ to 4½ years of age. It is during this period of changing teeth that most horses and mules are broken or trained and first used for hard work. The changing of teeth, especially when the temporary molars fail to shed and become firmly fixed caps on the crowns of the emerging permanent molars, is accompanied by pain and poor mastication. This trouble, combined with hard work, causes many colts to lose weight rapidly, appear unthrifty, and sometimes develop digestive disturbances (colic) if attention is not given to the teeth. Any unusual occurrence during feeding, such as slobbering, excessive drooling of saliva, sudden cessation of eating, or dropping of food from the mouth, is a symptom indicative of tooth trouble and should be investigated by a thorough examination of the animal's mouth.

The commonest disorders of horses' teeth are alveolar periostitis and uneven teeth.

Alveolar Periostitis and Uneven Teeth

The spaces occupied by the teeth in the jawbones are known as alveoli. The embedded part of the tooth is attached to the alveolus, or socket, by a layer of tissue known as the alveolar periosteum, an inflammation of which results in alveolar periostitis, which may extend to the dental pulp (the central, soft, gelatinous part of the tooth). Alveolar periostitis is usually caused by food particles and infective material which have gained entrance to the alveoli from the mouth. The food particles and the resulting decomposed infective material in the majority of cases enter the dental pulp from the grinding surface of the molars through improperly closed structures (infundibula) between the grinding surface and the pulp cavity. Infection may also be admitted through imperfect gums, through the spaces between the teeth, or through the exposure of the alveolar periosteum at the time of shedding the temporary molars. Occasionally the disease may result from cystic tumors, nutritional disturbances, or mechanical violence. The progressive involvement

---

4 The 4 canine (bridle) teeth found in the male are absent or very rudimentary in the mare. The so-called wolf teeth, which sometimes appear one on each side just in front of the first upper grinders, are vestiges of the first premolar teeth of the prehistoric horse.

of structures is always accompanied by an extremely offensive odor and more or less pain and difficulty in mastication. Abscesses may form deep in the sockets, involving the bony tissues, and may break through, discharging their contents through the skin on the lower jaw or into the sinuses of the upper jaw. In the latter case there may be a nasal discharge, Obstruction of the blood supply may occur and result in desiccation and often splitting of the tooth. Involvement of neighboring teeth and expulsion of the originally infected tooth may also occur.

The fourth superior (upper) molar is most often involved. The fifth and third superior and fourth inferior (lower) molars are less frequently affected, and the remaining molars rarely. The treatment indicated is early extraction under proper anesthesia.

The horse, like other herbivorous animals, has teeth that are specially adapted for intensive wear and differ from those of other animals and man. In the latter groups, the root only is embedded in the bony alveolus, and crown being fully exposed except where covered by the margins of the gums. In herbivorous animals, the crown is for the most part embedded in the bone in young animals, continuing its growth with wear. In extreme old age, even the true root may come into wear.

Enamel and dentine of unequal hardness make up the tooth surface; the latter being softer wears faster and produces the necessary rough grinding surface. When the grinding surfaces of the teeth of old animals have become smooth, the deep portion of the molars with little enamel has come into wear, and the animals should be fed ground or crushed feeds.

The distance between the two rows of upper grinders is greater than that between the rows of lower grinders. The grinding table of the upper molars is beveled downward toward the cheek and the opposing table of the lower molars slopes upward toward the tongue. This arrangement is well adapted to the lateral movement used by the horse in chewing its coarse feed. In the normal mouth the outer edge of the upper molars and the inner edge of the lower molars are quite sharp. Not infrequently these edges become excessively sharp or jagged and cause considerable injury to the cheeks and tongue, interfering with normal mastication. Such abnormalities may be corrected by appropriate rasping, or so-called floating.

When one or more teeth in a row in either jaw project or extend beyond the normal grinding plane, uneven wear results. This may lead to serious injury to the animal's mouth and cause improper mastication, followed by indigestion, malnutrition, and in the later stages general unthriftiness, loss of strength and emaciation.

Where the jaw protrudes, the first or last molars may become longer than others in the arcade because of failure to meet normal grinding opposition. The unopposed teeth continue to lengthen until they meet and injure the opposite gum. Likewise when a tooth is missing in an arcade, its opponent tends to elongate. Such abnormal teeth should be cut off to the level of the adjoining teeth at intervals, usually about once a year.

Occasionally the wolf teeth may cause irritation of the gums, and since they serve no useful purpose they may be extracted with benefit.

Fistula of the Withers and Poll Evil

Fistula of the withers is a general term loosely applied to any chronic, deep-seated inflammation in the region of the withers, usually accompanied by infection. The conditions included under this general heading are inflammation of the ligament (dorsal ceivical desmitis), aseptic or septic inflammation of the protective sheath above the spines of the vertebrae (dorsal bursitis), and true fistula of the withers, in which there is infection of all the structures previously mentioned and possibly the ends of the vertebral spines, with one or. more external discharging tracts.

There are differences of opinion among authorities as to the cause of fistula of the withers. It is thought by some that injury from blows, contact with feed racks or low doors, or collar pressure may start the inflammation. *Filaria labiato papillosa,* which is an almost invisible threadlike worm, has been recovered from the diseased tissues in numerous cases and is considered by some as the primary cause. In recent years, bacteriological investigations have revealed the presence of another possible cause, *Brucella abortus,* the germ responsible for brucellosis (Bang's disease) in cattle and for undulant fever in man.

Cervical desmitis frequently results from a slipping of the collar on the top part of the neck and may be controlled in the early stages by properly fitting the collar and adjusting the hame tugs at the center of pull on the shoulder. In more advanced cases surgical removal of the diseased part of the ligament and establishment of adequate drainage are essential for recovery.

The control of aseptic supra spinous bursitis, another primary stage of fistula of the withers, should include the removal of factors that may be responsible for external injury such as low feed racks, low doors, and rocks in the paddock where the animals roll. Conservative treatment is usually tried before resorting to the more drastic surgical procedure. The affected area may be shaved and painted with tincture of iodine or some other mild irritant. Internal medication may hasten and favor resorption in some cases. The use of any surgical instrument, such as a knife or needle, in a case of this type is to be avoided except under strictly aseptic conditions.

In those cases in which the contents of the bursea (sac) are septic or where a true fistula is present, the more radical surgical procedure is indicated. Removal of diseased tissue, including all the diseased tracts and pockets, and the establishment of drainage are essential before healing can be complete. Bacterins prepared from cultures of the micro-organisms found in individual cases are now being used experimentally. Control measures include all those previously mentioned in addition to blood testing for brucellosis. A positive blood test would indicate possible *Brucella* infection, the control of which in cattle and swine may help to eliminate the development of future cases.

Poll evil (atlantal bursitis) is a condition similar to fistula of the withers, differing only in that it affects the poll rather than the withers. The anatomical structures, elementary causes, and general methods for control and treatment are essentially the same.

Diseases Connected with Mismanagement

While most diseases of horses and mules are influenced indirectly in their occurrence and development by various methods of management of the animals, some are so directly connected with certain practices that it may be correctly said that they are caused by the practices in question.

The ailments here discussed include azoturia, heaves, colic, founder, collar and saddle sores, and certain forms of poisoning. In most of these, mismanagement, whether through ignorance, carelessness, or intention, is the direct cause.

Azoturia (Black Water, Monday-Morning Disease)

Azoturia is a specific disease of the horse, found most frequently in animals of draft type and characterized by sudden stiffening and paralysis of the muscles, usually in the hind legs, profuse sweating, and black or coffee-colored urine. It usually appears shortly after exercise is begun after a day or more of idleness. It occurs chiefly in animals that are receiving full feed and are in good condition and appears most frequently in the spring months.

Numerous theories have been presented concerning the specific cause. Originally the disease was named in the belief, since disproved, that it was due to an excess of nitrogenous substances in the urine. A plausible explanation is based on the lactic acid theory, developed in recent years. Lactic acid is one of the by products resulting from the metabolism of glycogen (animal starch) in the muscles. This natural process is accelerated before and during azoturia, according to some investigators. Excessive lactic acid is thought to cause deranged muscular activity, circulatory sluggishness, and muscular exhaustion. A working animal stores a large amount of glycogen in the muscles during a period of idleness, especially if it is kept on full feed, particularly on a high carbohydrate diet. Such an animal may develop an excess of lactic acid in the muscle tissue when returned to work, with consequent danger of azoturia.

Control measures consist in regulation of the diet during rest periods–cutting the ration to a minimum and giving laxative feeds such as bran–and, if possible, allowing the animals to exercise naturally in a paddock.

All animals should be closely watched when resuming work after a lay-off. If the disease develops, successful treatment requires immediate, absolute rest, in a standing position if possible. This means that the animal should not be moved from the spot where it becomes affected unless absolutely necessary, and then by truck or similar means. Such a procedure may require the erection of a temporary shelter, as well as slings for supporting the animal. Medication must vary with the severity of the case, and veterinary service is essential to determine the necessity of sedatives, laxatives, alkalizing drugs etc., and to advise on the general care of the animal. A large percentage of affected animals that have been down for some time before the beginning of treatment are lost in spite of the best possible care.

Heaves (Broken Wind, Asthma)

Heaves is a chronic respiratory disease of the horse characterized by difficult breathing and a dry, wheezing cough, resulting finally in emphysema (infiltration of air into the tissues) of the lung.

While the exact cause is unknown, recent studies indicate that the condition is especially apt to follow chronic inflammatory conditions of the lungs, chiefly bronchitis. Authorities agree that the main source of trouble is associated with the feeding of damaged roughage. The condition very seldom develops in pastured animals or those fed corn fodder or clean hay, but it occurs commonly in animals fed dusty or moldy hay, made from either legumes or grasses. The inhalation of dust from such hay aggravates any respiratory trouble that may be present and is especially provocative in established cases of pulmonary emphysema.

In the respiration characteristic of heaves there is a double lift of the flank, and exhalation of air requires special muscular effort. The symptoms are increased by hard or fast work, large draughts of cold water, sudden changes in weather, protracted heat or cold, and overfeeding, especially of roughages. change from clean, bright hay to poorer quality feed often aggravates the condition.

There is no specific remedy, although certain arsenic and other tonics are said to be beneficial in some cases. In advanced cases nothing can be done to overcome the extensive pulmonary abnormality. The symptoms in milder cases can be controlled by feeding only sound hay, preferably in a quantity less than is normally given, with the grain ration increased if necessary. Some affected animals improve markedly if they are placed on pasture for several months or if only light work, alternated with periods of pasturing, is given. If questionable fodder must be used, it should be fed in as limited a quantity as possible under individual conditions. Sprinkling the fodder lightly with water will serve to lessen the likelihood of inhalation of dust.

Colic

The term "colic" is commonly used for abdominal pain and associated symptoms resulting from anyone of numerous disorders of the abdominal cavity. In this discussion, acute dilatation of the stomach, tympany (bloat), impaction (stoppage), obstipation (extreme constipation), intestinal obstruction, torsion (twist or gut tie), strangulation, gastrointestinal catarrh, gastroenteritis, and thromboembolic colic, either alone or in combination with one another, are considered.

The most common conditions are acute dilatation or overloading of the stomach, tympany, and impaction of the large intestines and cecum. These conditions are primarily disorders of function without complicating organic changes of the tissues, which may follow, however, if the condition is not relieved. Some functional digestive disturbances may occur unavoidably as a result of organic disease. However, the majority of colic cases are the result of faulty management, especially improper feeding and poor feed. A functional disturbance of one part of the digestive tract, such as that caused by overloading the stomach, may result in rapid involvement of the entire tract. Thus, stasis (atony, or discontinued muscular movements) of the intestines, followed by fermentation (gas formation), obstipation, and autointoxication, finally terminating in organic changes such as catarrh, inflammation, edema, and hemorrhage, may occur.

Some of the more common causes of digestive disturbances are change of feed, overeating, idleness on a full-work diet; fatigue, excessive drinking, defective teeth, greedy eating, spoiled or fibrous indigestible feed, exposure to abrupt changes in weather, and overwork. Sudden change of feed, either of grain or roughage, will invariably cause indigestion in some horses. Though others are less sensitive to a change, it is always good practice to make feed changes, gradually over a period of several days. Overeating, resulting from gaining access to the grain bin; a new field, or some other source of unlimited feed, causes acute dilatation of the stomach and intestines. Work animals standing idle on full feed often develop indigestion as a result of intestinal stasis, faulty elimination, and autointoxication.

Fatigue, exhaustion, and overwork cause a reflex paralysis of the digestive system, making animals more susceptible to digestive disturbances. This condition occurs most frequently in the spring when the horses are first put to heavy work and their feed is increased. The trouble may be avoided in many instances by starting the grain ration 5 or 6 weeks before the heavy work begins. The ration should be increased gradually with an increase in exercise, green animals being worked only part time until they are thoroughly hardened.

Excessive drinking after heavy work is frequently followed by symptoms of indigestion. Water should be withheld until the animal has "cooled out." Two or three swallows of water at a time may safely be allowed at frequent intervals during the cooling process.

Defective teeth cause faulty mastication, which may result in improper digestion and absorption of food, followed by general unthriftiness. The teeth should be examined regularly and defects corrected.

Indigestion from greedy eating parallels symptoms from defective teeth because of improper mastication and in addition frequently produces choke–stoppage of the esophagus (gullet). Complications from this condition predispose to other disorders. Stones or coarse wire mesh in the animal's feed box will decrease the amount of food he can take in his mouth and usually force him to eat with less haste.

Feeds that are moldy, sour, filthy, frozen, improperly cured, full of dirt or dust, fibrous, and indigestible are always dangerous.

Exposure during cold, wet, and stormy weather has proved favorable for the development of colic due to reflex digestive paralysis, increased hunger, frozen feeds, and insufficient intake of water. It is a good practice following exposure to rub the animal dry arid then give a little water and hay, withholding grain for an hour or two.

Treatment of colic is as variable as the numerous disorders discussed under that name because of the many causes and the different courses the disease may take. It is advisable to get veterinary assistance during the early stages. To reduce danger from falling, kicking, or rolling, the animal should be placed in a large, deeply bedded box stall or moved out of the stable with an attendant. A slow walk will often keep an animal from injuring itself during severe pain and sometimes may help to ease the pain. The giving of drenches, especially through the nose, by inexperienced laymen is inadvisable because of the danger of strangulation, which may be followed by sudden death or mechanical pneumonia. Today most veterinarians use the stomach tube in the treatment of colic. This not only affords immediate relief of most acute stomach colics through the escape of accumulated gas, but it permits washing out the stomach and in addition eliminates the hazards of drenching.

Founder (Lamenitis)

Laminitis, or founder, is a serious ailment of the fleshy laminae of the horse's feet which commonly follows heavy overfeeding, chiefly on grains, and also gorging on green plants or any feed so palatable that excessive amounts are consumed. Other causes, such as metritis (inflammation of the uterus) in recently foaled mares long-continued, or hard, fast work on hard footing, or general intoxication (poisoning) may be responsible, but overeating is the principal cause.

Extreme pain and fever (103°-106° F.) are the chief symptoms. Affected animals are very reluctant to move, and when they are compelled to do so there is excrutiating pain as shown by a peculiar crouching gait, indications of anxiety, and trembling. In most cases all four feet are more or less involved, although it may be evident mostly in the front feet, in which case they are extended in front of the body with the weight on the heels. If the hind feet only are involved, all four feet are bunched under the body, the forefeet and the heels of the hind feet supporting the weight. A severe injury in one leg may lead to laminitis in the foot of the opposite side. The affected feet are hot and throbbing, and the arteries along the pastern can be felt with unusual ease. The slightest pressure on the foot causes the animal to snatch it quickly from the ground.

The first principle of treatment is to place the feet in a cold foot bath, with ice if it is available. The attendant can do this pending the arrival of the veterinarian. Prompt purgation is an important part of the treatment in cases due to gorging. In many cases hypodermic medication is indicated. This is one of the few ailments of animals which may be improved by bleeding, but even here bleeding is not applicable to every case. With prompt and proper treatment; the acute symptoms usually begin to subside in a few days, unless complications arise, which may cause death.

Chronic laminitis results in more or less irremediable deformity of the foot. The hoof wall develops deep rings, and the sole drops. Except for suitable shoeing, little can be done in the way of treatment.

Collar and Saddle Sores

Certain sores must be attributed primarily to poor conditioning of the animal and to an improperly fitted or poorly adjusted collar or saddle. Either a bruise or chafing of the skin when continually irritated leads to the formation of so-called galls, or sitfasts. These consist of necrotic tissue combined with dense fibrous tissue. Any such lesion may be complicated by the presence of infection.

To prevent these sores, the animals should be gradually hardened to work. This conditioning, together with thorough and regular grooming and properly fitted equipment, is usually all that is required.

If sores do form and work is continued, surgical removal with a period of rest for healing usually becomes necessary. Sometimes with a period of rest the newly formed callouses may slough off or become largely resorbed.

Poisoning

Aside from the poisoning due to eating certain plants and the intoxications considered in connection with encephalomyelitis, both of which are discussed elsewhere, the chief source of poisoning in horses and mules is the consumption of such common toxic substances as arsenic and lead.

Carelessness in handling arsenical preparations such as grasshopper bait, paris green, and other plant sprays, as well as arsenical dips, is usually the cause of arsenic poisoning in horses and mules, though injudicious administration of arsenical drugs is sometimes responsible.

When large quantities of arsenicals are consumed the symptoms are usually acute. There is a sudden onset of trembling, restlessness, increased thirst, rapid breathing, colic, prostration, staggering, and extreme sickness. In most cases death follows in 2 or 3 hours. Chronic cases result from the consumption of a smaller amount of arsenic over a period of weeks and may show unthriftiness, rough coat, garlic breath, raised red gum lines, lazy action, easy tiring, and partial paralysis of the hind legs. Treatment in acute cases is often Ineffective because of the large amount of arsenic consumed and the rapid course of the disease. Animals that have recently consumed the poison should have the stomach contents removed with a stomach tube and circulatory stimulants and peripheral nerve depressants administered. The most valuable antidote is sodium hyposulfite given by mouth or in the blood stream or both. If the veterinarian is not readily available, as much as a handful of the salt may be given in a drench.

Lead, like arsenic, combines with other elements to form various salts, the most common of which are lead acetate (sugar of lead), red oxide of lead, white lead, lead oxide, and arsenate of lead. The toxic salts of lead have a wide variety of uses in agriculture and are made available to animals by careless use of such substances as sprays, dusting powders, and paints.

Acute lead poisoning does not occur in equines as commonly as, in cattle. The symptoms are usually those of indigestion, accompanied by a partial paralysis (knuckling of the joints). Chronic lead poisoning has been commonly observed in districts where small amounts of lead may continually be taken into the body through feed, water, or inhaled lead dust. Such districts are found around lead mines, smelters, and orchards or fields where much spraying is done.

The first noticeable symptom of chronic poisoning is some form of paralysis, usually laryngeal, or throat, made apparent by "choking down," or roaring, following exercise. The time necessary for symptoms to develop varies from several months to as long as a few years, depending on the amount of poison and the rate of Intake.

Control may be exercised by giving particular attention to keeping animals away from the source of the poison. Feed may be brought in from outside the dangerous districts, water should be frequently tested for lead, and both feed and water should be protected against further contamination from lead sprays or dust. Muzzles may be placed on horses to prevent their eating vegetable matter while working in sprayed orchards and fields.

In districts where horses are continuously exposed to lead and develop chronic poisoning, animals that become unserviceable may be removed to an uncontaminated environment before the disease has progressed too far. Often such animals will recover sufficiently to do general farm work.

During the convalescent period, various forms of medication may be helpful. When the laryngeal paralysis does not improve, it is a more or less common practice to insert a trachea tube, which often enables the animal to do moderate work without difficulty in breathing. In such cases the tube and the opening must be cleaned frequently.

Acute lead poisoning may be treated by administering the chemical antidotes, dilute sulfuric acid, magnesium sulfate, or sodium sulfate, which combine with lead to form insoluble lead salts. Stimulants for paralysis, protective for inflamed stomach and intestines, and other treatment should be administered when necessary.

Chapter 7

INTERNAL PARASITES OF HORSES AND MULES

Aurel O. Foster[1]

[1] *Aurel O. Foster is Associate Parasitologist, Zoological Division, Bureau of Animal Industry.*

Some 150 kinds of internal parasites infest horses and mules, and probably no individual animal is ever entirely free of some of them. Fortunately, comparatively few do real damage–but those few can be extremely harmful and sometimes deadly. Here are the facts about a complicated subject.

The domestic equines provide shelter and subsistence to approximately 150 kinds of protozoa and worms which live as internal parasites.[2] There are few horse owners who have not had some first-hand experience with many of these, and nearly everyone is familiar, in one way or another, with at least some of them. Among the protozoa are the blood-inhabiting trypanosomes and piroplasmata, the ciliates of the large bowel, and several miscellaneous species. The parasitic worms include flukes, tapeworms, stomach worms, large roundworms, strongyles, pinworms, lungworms, filariae, and some others.

---

[2] Horse bots as internal parasites of horses and mules are discussed in another article in this volume.

Some of the worst diseases of equines are caused by these invaders; yet they do not, as a rule, cause specific and spectacular diseases. In every case of harmful parasitism, the damaging effects are essentially of two kinds–general and specific. The general effect, although seldom as obvious, is unquestionably more important than the specific effect from an economic standpoint. It always causes a loss in the functional efficiency of the animal as a working unit. In some instances, as in such a disease as dourine, the specific effects, clinical or pathological or both, definitely indicate the disease. In most cases., however, as best typified, perhaps, by strongylosis, the specific effects are subordinated to the net general effect of the parasitism–decreased efficiency. Symptoms in such cases are manifold, but so variable as to preclude definite, diagnosis.

The full importance of parasitism is inadequately understood. The parasite itself is ordinarily dealt with as the, agent of disease or debility, but it is possible that parasites play some role in the transmission of other serious diseases, provide portals of entry for harmful micro-organisms, or serve as reservoirs of infection for other diseases. Moreover, parasites may be capable in themselves of exerting effects which have not hitherto been noted. Investigations along these lines have only begun.

Equines everywhere appear to be infected with internal parasites. There are, however, important differences in degree and kind of parasitism in different parts of the world and among individual horses and mules. Fortunately, several of the more pathogenic, or disease-producing, species, such as the blood-inhabiting protozoa, are limited in their distribution and incidence. The intestinal protozoa, however, occur everywhere and possibly in every horse and mule. The most numerous of these are the ciliated forms that live chiefly in the colon. They can be detected readily by microscopic examination of a watered drop of fresh manure. Some of the parasitic worms are distributed more or less regionally but as, there are so many kinds of them and they are so unrelated, it is, difficult to make any general statement about them. Most of the important nematodes, too, particularly the strongyles, are found wherever there are equines, and it is doubtful whether any horse or mule is entirely free of them, except perhaps for a short period after an efficient anthelmintic has been administered.

Differences in distribution are probably determined, in general, by differences in developmental cycles. For example, the distribution of species which require intermediate hosts for transmission is more limited than that of species which are able to develop during a short period in the open. Also contributing to the distribution of equine parasites is the fact that horses and mules, perhaps more than other domestic animals, have been transported, widely for service in war and in colonizing enterprises and for racing and breeding purposes.

Some of the parasites–most of the trypanosomes, for example–are capable of infecting a wide range of mammals, but the majority are so specialized that they can exist only in equine hosts. Some species, indeed, are better adapted to horses and mules than to donkeys, and others prefer donkeys to other equines. In general, horses and mules appear to be about equally susceptible to most parasites, although some kinds, such as the trypanosomes, are more injurious to horses than to mules.

Within their hosts these parasitic organisms exhibit a high degree of adaptability to specific locations. Most of them normally parasitize the alimentary tract, lungs, body cavity, or blood stream. In the alimentary tract, however some species are exclusively parasites of the stomach, others of the small intestine, and others of the large, intestine. Moreover, the several species of strongyles which inhabit the large bowel tend to become localized in specific parts of this organ–the cecum, the ventral colon. or the dorsal colon. In addition to the parasites thus localized, several of the species follow various migratory circuits within the host, whereas many are aberrant, or wandering, in their habits. Consequently, scarcely apart or organ of an animal is entirely free from potential parasitic invasion. Thus there are parasites of horses and mules that live on the surface of the body; in the nose, ears, and eyes; in the skin, muscles, ligaments, visceral organs, or body cavity; or elsewhere in the body. It will also become evident from the following discussions that a parasite which in its adult stage normally inhabits one region of the body may, in its immature stages, be responsible for serious injury in an entirely different part.

Protozoan Parasites

Except for a few species, the protozoa of equines fall into two groups, those that inhabit the blood and those that live in the large bowel. All the important disease-producing agents are in the first group. The latter group embraces a large number of species that are essentially innocuous and may, in some instances, be actually beneficial to their hosts. In general the former require an intermediate host for their transmission or have an otherwise complicated life history, whereas the latter follow a simple, direct developmental cycle. Those of the blood-inhabiting group are chiefly trypanosomes and piroplasmata, which fortunately have a relatively limited distribution. Although herds have been decimated by infection with these organisms, the incidence of infection is usually not high, even in endemic areas, where cases of infection are always present. In contrast, the latter group–those inhabiting the large bowel–is composed principally of ciliates, which are believed to occur in all equines everywhere.

Trypanosome Diseases

The trypanosomes are by far the most important protozoan parasites of equines. They cause such diseases as dourine, surra, nagana, mal de caderas, and miurrina, each of which takes a heavy toll among the equine populations of regions where it has become established.

Dourine is the only one of these trypanosome diseases that occurs in the United States. It is caused by *Trypanosoma equiperdum* and is widely distributed. It differs from other trypanosome infections in that it is essentially chronic rather than acute and is transmitted directly from horse to horse, usually during coitus, without the assistance of an insect or mammalian vector.

Surra, caused by *Trypanosoma evansi*, is the oldest recorded trypanosome disease of equines. It is an acute, usually fatal, infection, running its course generally within a few weeks. It occurs chiefly in central and southern Asia and in the Philippines. Horseflies (*Tabanus* species) are thought to be the chief vectors, although the method of spread is purely mechanical.

The disease nagana is prevalent in east and central Africa and floes not occur elsewhere. The commonest agent of the infection is *Trypanosoma burcei*, a variety of which is the cause of Rhodesian sleeping sickness of man. In equines the disease is usually fatal in a few weeks, being too acute for the characteristic manifestations of sleeping sickness. It is carried from horse to horse by tsetse flies, in which the trypanosome completes a definite cycle of development.

Mal de caderas is related to surra and may be identical with it. It differs from typical surra, however, in the apparent morphology (form and structure) of its causative agent, *Trypanosoma equinum*, and in its distribution. It occurs only in South America and is believed to be transmitted by horseflies and stableflies.

Murrina, like mal de caderas, is similar to surra, and its causative agent, *Trypanosoma hippicum*, is closely related to *T. evansi*. The disease occurs chiefly in Panama, where it is transmitted, at least in part, by bloodsucking vampire bats. Affected animals, if untreated, usually die in a few weeks or months.

Piroplasmosis

Piroplasmosis, also known as tick fever, biliary fever, and hemoglobinuric fever, is an acute febrile condition characterized by jaundice, hemoglobinuria (hemoglobin in the urine), and anemia. It is caused by the presence of microscopic organisms, known as piroplasms of piroplasmata, in the red blood cells. In important respects it is like tick fever of cattle, but it does not occur in the United States, The majority of cases apparently recover, some within a few days or weeks, but the blood usually remains infective for several months or even years. Unlike the trypanosome infections, piroplasmosis confers a reasonably durable immunity. *Nuttallia equi*, the commonest agent of equine piroplasmosis, occurs in Africa, Southern Europe, Transcaucasla, Southern Asia, and South America. In Africa, it is transmitted by ticks belonging to the genus *Rhipicephalus*. Another species of the organism, *Babesia caballi*, occurs along with *Nuttallia equi* in Italy, India, and Macedonia, and is also found in Russia, Transcaucasia, North Africa, and Panama. This organism also is transmitted by ticks, chiefly species of *Dermacentor* and *Boophilus*.

Intestinal Ciliates and Other Protozoa

At least 50 species of ciliated intestinal protozoa, belonging to half as many genera, are common inhabitants of the large bowel of equines. There is no acceptable evidence that they cause disease; indeed various investigators have now and then advanced the hypothesis that these organisms perform some useful service for their hosts. They may, for example, assist the digestive functions by breaking down certain otherwise indigestible materials into substances that can be readily assimilated. Millions of these organisms pass out every day with the feces of an infected animal.

In spite of their universal presence in equines and their striking variety and abundance, the method of transmission of ciliated intestinal protozoa has not been satisfactorily explained. It is assumed that new hosts are infected by swallowing living organisms in contaminated food and drink, although it is recognized that such organisms, after entering by the mouth, would require certain adaptations in order to reach the cecum or colon.

Besides trypanosomes, piroplasmata, and ciliates, several miscellaneous species of protozoa occur in domestic equines, some more or less commonly. Among these are the muscle-infecting sarcosporidia, plasmodial parasites of the blood similar to those causing human malaria, flagellates, and Suctoria of the intestine of interest are three species of amoebae that are analogous to three similar species occurring in man. They are *Endamoeba gedoelsti* (syn. *E. intestinalis*), the large and presumably harmless amoeba of the colon, comparable to *E. coli* of man; *E. equi*, a smaller colon amoeba; allegedly disease producing, suggesting the form parasitic in man, *E. histolytica*; and *E. gingivalis* var. *equi*, the equine variety of the human oral amoeba. About these very little is known, and only after further study can their importance be evaluated.

Helminthic Parasites

The helminths, or worm parasites, of equines are more varied and numerous than are the parasitic protozoa, and economically they are immeasurably more important. In contrast to the specific and fatal diseases caused by certain of the protozoa, the damage caused by worms is usually not spectacular; sometimes it is scarcely apparent, and rarely is it an immediate cause of death. Moreover, the symptoms are usually too general to serve for diagnosis. The important net effect of worm parasitism in equines is reduced efficiency. Judged on that basis, it becomes as obvious as it is paradoxical that parasites which kill their host animals are frequently of less economic significance than are those which insidiously undermine their efficiency.

Horse Strongyles and Strongylosis

The horse strongyles are a large, unified group of approximately 40 species belonging to a single nematode, family, the strongylidae.

Most of them are relatively small, less than an inch in length; some are scarcely visible to the unaided eye. These are commonly known as small strongyles, cylicostomes, or *Trichonema* species. A few strongyles are large, as much as 2 inches long, and are usually firmly attached within the host and sucking blood. The front third of these larger worms frequently contains fresh blood, which gives that part a red color in contrast to the hind portion, which is darker and more or less slate-colored. There are three species of the genus Strongylus, which are variously referred to as large strongyles, sclerostomes, palisade worms, red worms, and blood worms. Undoubtedly the widespread economic importance of these parasites largely accounts for the variety of common names applied to them.

All the strongyles have broadly, similar developmental cycles. During their adult life, they live in the large bowel and tend to become localized in one or another part of this relatively limited portion of the digestive tract. The females deposit large numbers of eggs, which leave the host's body with the feces. The eggs can, and probably normally do, develop and hatch while in the bolus of feces. Unlike the eggs of many parasitic nematodes of other hosts, they do not appear to be delayed or inhibited in their development until the feces are diluted with rain water, earth, or some other agent. This adaptation probably protects the eggs and larvae from the damaging effects of such natural factors as sunlight, desiccation, and cold. Embryonic development is rapid, and the first-stage larvae usually hatch during the second day. In 6 to 10 days, the larvae molt twice and become third-stage, infective larvae. The second sheath is retained, probably as further protection against the hazards of an unfavorable environment. First- and second-stage larvae die rapidly when subjected to drying, marked heat or cold, or excessive bacterial action, but the infective larvae may survive for months or even years under these conditions. The infective larvae rest on the upper, more accessible portions of grass blades and are usually swallowed by horses during grazing. Once swallowed, they undergo a developmental cycle within the host many aspects of which are not yet perfectly understood.

Present evidence indicates that the large and small strongyles have certain essential differences in their cycles of migration and development within the host. The large strongyles migrate extensively within the host, and their migrations are associated with some of the most serious aspects of strongylosis. Moreover, it is becoming increasingly evident that the wanderings of the larvae of the three large strongyles take them to different localities in the host's body–*Strongylus equinus* to the pancreas, *S. edentatus* to the lining membranes and visceral supporting tissue of the body cavity, and *S. vulgalris* to the walls of the visceral arteries.

The small strongyles are believed to pass directly to the large intestine, where at least some of them penetrate the mucous membrane and settle down in the intestinal wall for a period of growth. It is doubtful whether all the cylicostomes undergo this tissue stage, since at autopsy fourth and fifth-stage worms can usually be found both in the cavity of the intestine and encysted in the mucosa.

The palisade worms and their close relatives differ from the cylicostomes also in their mode of life within the large intestine. Most of the palisade worms attach themselves tenaciously to the mucosa and live as bloodsuckers; the cylicostomes, although capable of attachment, are usually found free in the lumen, but on the surface of the fecal mass in close contact with the intestinal lining.

It becomes apparent from what has been said that strongylosis is not a simple condition of parasitism. The bloodsucking activities of the adult large strongyles produce anemia which in turn gives rise to many of the symptoms that ordinarily accompany severe strongylosis. By shifting their points of attachment, these parasites leave minute hemorrhages and denuded areas which are favorable sites for bacterial colonization. In their larval stages, they cause transient inflammatory and irritative changes throughout the viscera. Many of these ultimately become scars, adhesions, or caseous (cheese-like) nodules. The larvae of *Strongylus vulgaris* cause dilation and obstruction of blood vessels. Colic is a frequent result of the decreased blood supply to the intestine, and verminous inflammation of the inner wall of an artery always impairs the capacity for arduous work. Intermittent lameness is believed to result often from stoppage of the smaller leg arteries occasioned by the liberation of clotted particles from within a tumor of a blood vessel. Sometimes the wall of the vessel ruptures, causing sudden death by internal hemorrhage.

Animals with severe strongylosis exhibit lack of appetite, anemia, and progressive emaciation. The body wall has a tucked-in appearance, and the animal loses condition generally.

The diagnosis of strongylosis is not easy. The presence of the characteristic ova in the feces is evidence of strongylid infestation, but not necessarily an indication of disease. Most horses in reasonable good condition pass a few of these ova. In general, however, a high concentration of strongyle eggs in the feces, combined with loss of condition and an absence of organic or infectious disease, is strong presumptive evidence of strongylosis.

Not all the 40 different kinds of strongyles have ever been found in anyone horse or mule, but every animal almost invariably harbors. several of them. It is, therefore, legitimate to ask how many kinds of strongyles occur in the average horse and what are the more or less average maximum and minimum numbers. Study of a considerable body of literature indicates that, qualitatively, strongyle infections of equines vary only slightly in different parts of the world and that, quantitatively, the average horse or mule harbors from one-fourth to one-half of the known strongylid species. One or more of the three species of large strongyles are usually present, along with 10 to 12 species of small strongyles. It appears that about 15 species account for the bulk of strongylid parasitism in equines and that the other 25 do not occur in significant numbers.

The characteristic strongyles occurring in the cecum of horses and mules may be said to be *Strongylus vulgaris*, *S. equinus*, *Cyathostomim coronatum*, *Cylicostephanus calicatus*, and *Cylicocyclus nassatus*. The majority of the strongylid fauna in the ventral colon are of the following species: *Cylicocyclus nassatus*, *Cylicostephanus minutus*, *C. calicatus*, *Cylicocercus catinatus*, *C. pateratus*, *Cyathostomum labiatum*, *C. labratum*, *Triodontophorus minor*, and *Strongylus edentatus*. The typical fauna of the dorsal colon are *Cylicostephanus longibursatus*, *Cylicocyclus insignie*, *C. nassatus*, *Cylicocercus goldi*, and *C. catinatus*.

Of the 36,000 strongyles recovered in one study, it was found that approximately four-fifths were accounted for by fewer than one-fifth of the species, the six commonest–*Cylicocyclus nassatus*, *C. insigne*, *Cylicostephanus longibursatus*, *C. calicatus*, *C. minutus*, and *Strongylus vulgaris*–which are of the greatest economic importance.

Data from several studies suggest that equines harboring approximately 1,000 strongyles are lightly infected; that infections of 30,000 to 50,000 are not infrequent and probably do not as a rule produce symptoms; but that infections of over 50,000 are relatively severe and may result in more or less typical strongylosis.

Both the degree and, to a less extent, the kind of parasitism are affected by many factors, some of which it is possible to evaluate to a limited extent. For example, the size of worm infestations depends principally upon the extent of exposure to infection, and this is influenced by conditions of sanitation, feeding, medication, season, and climate. In addition, observational evidence has demonstrated that infections are more severe in younger animals. There are also certain apparent host "preferences" among the strongylids. *Cyathostomum tetracanthum*, *Cylicocyclus auriculatus*, and *C. elongatus* are characteristically found in donkeys and are relatively rare in horses and mules. *Cylicocercus alveatus* and *Cylicocyclus triramosus* are common only in zebras, but are more often found in donkeys that in horses or mules. *Cylicostephanus poculatus*, typically found in horses, has been recorded once from a mule but never from donkeys or zebras. There is evidence also that some breeds of horses are probably more resistant to intestinal parasites than are others.

Other Helminths and the Diseases Caused by Them

Besides the strongyles, several more or less unrelated helminths, some of which are of considerable economic importance, affect equines. They are the flukes, tapeworms, stomach worms, ascarids, Strongyloides, pinworms, lungworms, and filariae.

Flukes

About a dozen species of trematodes, or flukes, have been reported, though not frequently, from the liver, blood vessels, and alimentary tract of horses and mules. Probably none are normal parasites of these animals. Those most commonly found in equines are the well-known liver flukes of sheep and cattle (*Fasciola hepatica* and *F. gigantica*) and certain species of blood flukes, of which *Schistosoma indicum* is the most important. The last occurs in India and Rhodesia but not elsewhere so far as is known.

Tapeworms

About 10 species of cestodes, or tapeworms, have been found in,. equines, but only 3 are of economic importance. These are *Anoplocephala magna*, *A. perfoliata*; and *Paranoplocephala mamillana*.

The first is the largest of the horse tapeworms, although it seldom exceeds 10 inches in length. Its prominent head bears four conspicuous suckers, and the body is wide and tough. *Anoplocephala magna*, which occurs normally in the small intestine and rarely in the stomach or cecum, is the commonest tapeworm of American horses. Heavy infestations cause intestinal catarrh, with a consequent disturbance of digestive functions sometimes leading to emaciation and anemia.

The so-called lappetted tapeworm (*Anoplocephala perfoliata*) is 1 to 2 inches long and usually lives in the cecum, although it is sometimes encountered in the lower end of the small intestine. It is responsible for characteristic changes in the mucous membrane. The parasites tend to become localized in a small area immediately surrounding the opening of the small intestine into the cecum, the so-called ileocecal valve region. A hundred or more specimens may be encountered within an area with a diameter of 3 or 4 inches, their heads tenaciously attached and their bodies tightly packed against one another. At this site, the mucous membrane undergoes marked irritative and inflammatory changes, the most serious and conspicuous being a rapidly growing granular lesion. This mass, of growing tissue with its eroded surface is seldom larger than a tennis ball, but because of its location it progressively obstructs the ileocecal orifice. Sometimes, however, the process is one of making the tissue thinner rather than thicker, and this has led in some instances to perforation of the intestinal wall. Both processes result eventually in the death of the host animal. Although *A. perfoliata* is a widespread parasite of horses, its geographical occurrence is not well known. It appears to be relatively uncommon in continental United States, but it is the most frequently occurring horse tape-worm in some tropical countries, such as Panama and the Philippine Islands.

Paranoplocephala mamillana is known as the dwarf horse tapeworm. It seldom measures more than an inch in length and is relatively delicate. Although of widespread occurrence this tapeworm is seldom found in large numbers. It lives normally in the upper part of the small intestine and is of less economic significance than the two species already discussed.

The developmental cycles of the horse tapeworms have not been completely determined. The segments filled with eggs break off into the fecal mass, and the eggs are liberated either before or after the feces are deposited on the open ground. Judging from the recently determined cycles of a few related species of tapeworms, it appears probable that the eggs are ingested by arthropod intermediate hosts, perhaps certain pasture mites, in which the larval stages develop. This vector, in turn, is eaten by a grazing horse or mule.

Stomach Worms

Of some 9 or 10 kinds of parasitic worms that have been found in the stomachs of horses,. 4 are normally parasitic in these hosts and are the causative agents of a complex of lesions which gives rise to a serious condition known as verminous gastritis or inflammation of the stomach. Three of these worms are closely related and are known as *Habronema muscae, H. majus* (syn. *H. microstoma*), and *Draschia* (formerly *Habronema*) *megastoma*. They are transmitted by houseflies and small stableflies. The fourth species, *Trichostrongylus axei,* is more frequently a parasite of cattle, sheep, and goats than of equines and is so small that it may be overlooked at post mortem inspection unless a special search is made for it. *T. axei* does not require an intermediate host but infects the definitive host directly, after the manner of the strongyles.

Habronema muscae and *H. majus* are frequently seen on post mortem examination as slender, whitish worms actively whipping about in the stomach contents, especially if the contents are fluid or have been flushed out with water. The majority of specimens, however, live close to the glands of the stomach, embedded in mucus, or sometimes superficially embedded in the lining of the stomach. In this location it is sometimes difficult to discover them unless they are scraped or teased out. Horses harboring 200 or 300 worms generally have some inflammation of the lining of the stomach, and this contributes to gastric irritability, disordered digestion, and sometimes colic.

Draschia megastoma is less frequently found, but has more serious effects than the other species. These worms bury themselves deep in the mucous membrane and the layer beneath it and produce abscesses. Although such lesions are usually called tumors, they have, probably in every instance, a pus-filled or cheese-like core, in which are many worms and a cavernous tract communicating with the stomach. The tissue surrounding the central core shows marked thickening that gives the lesion a tumorous aspect. The diameter of the lesions varies from that of a walnut to that of an orange. Although these so-called tumors may occur in all areas of the glandular lining of the stomach, a preferred site is that portion nearest the border of the upper, nonglandular area. Not infrequently only a single abscess is present, although often there are many of various sizes. Because of their erosive nature, the abscesses produced by *D. megastoma* occasionally cause acute conditions, such as hemorrhage and perforation, but usually the injury is confined to irritative changes and more or less functional damage to the glandutar mucuous membrane.

The larvae of the larger stomach worms, especially those of the last-mentioned species, are responsible in part for a relatively common skin disease of horses called summer sores or bursati. Recently this condition has been increasingly referred to as cutaneous habronemiasis. Although the cause and development of this disease are imperfectly understood, available evidence indicates that the larvae are liberated when infected flies feed on skin wounds or sores. The immature worms in the head region of the fly probably escape by way of the fly's mouth when activated by the warmth of the horse's body. These larvae not only irritate the wounds and make them ugly in appearance but seem to prevent them from healing.

Trichostrongylus axei, the small stomach worm, is probably acquired by horses through association with ruminants. It is, however, a sufficiently important parasite of equines to have been considered by many investigators the principal cause of verminous inflammation of the stomach. Its mode of development is roughly similar to that of the strongyles, except that it does not wander in the body of the host and that it produces characteristic changes in the lining of the stomach. The worms are too small to be readily seen, but the infection can frequently be diagnosed on post mortem inspection by the character of the lesions. Not always, however, is infection with this species accompanied by grossly apparent lesions, and when such lesions are encountered, they may be of a varying nature. In general, stomachs infected with *T. axei* show a number of isolated, raised, button-like areas on the glandular mucosa. These may be the size of a dollar and depressed in the center, or they may be very small and inconspicuous. Sometimes the affected area is large and has a plateau-like appearance. In other cases the lesions are narrow at the base and somewhat mushroomed superficially. In all instances the disease process appears to be a progressive growth of tissue in response to irritative action by the worms.

Workers in both Europe and the United States have expressed the view that probably no other affection of equines is so regularly associated with a relatively sudden loss of condition.

The Large Roundworms, or Ascarids

The common roundworm, *Parascaris equorum,* is the largest parasite of equines. Female specimens vary from 6 to 15 inches in length; males, from 5 to 11 inches. When fully grown they have about the diameter of a lead pencil. They live in the small intestine and are typically parasitic in foals and young animals; only rarely are ascarids important in horses over 4 and 5 years of age, although a few specimens may be present in older animals.

The development cycle of the horse ascarid is simple except for a rather complicated migratory circuit within the host. Female worms in the small intestine deposit many eggs, which pass to the outside with the feces. If the weather is warm and the environment not excessively dry, the egg develop embryos and are infective to horses in about 2 weeks. When the infective eggs are swallowed by grazing horses, the embryos are liberated in the intestine. They rapidly penetrate the gut wall and are taken by the blood stream to the liver and thence through the heart to the lungs. In the lungs, usually about a week after infection, the larvae escape from the blood stream and migrate up the trachea to the pharynx. After being swallowed once more, the worms develop to maturity in the small intestine.

Because ascarids do not attach themselves to the intestinal mucous membranes they are sometimes considered to be relatively innocuous. In reality, however, they have three attributes which make them very dangerous:

(1) The migrations of the larvae through the liver and lungs cause extensive injury to these organs. In massive infections, serious inflammation of the liver or lungs may result.

(2) The large size of the adult worms makes heavy infections particularly injurious. In foals the presence of large numbers of ascarids is a fairly frequent cause of partial obstruction of the small intestine, and fatalities from complete obstruction or perforation have been recorded.

(3) The large roundworms tend to wander about in the intestine and, if the environment becomes unfavorable, to seek escape

through whatever channels are accessible. Cases are recorded of invasion and obstruction of the common bile duct and, more frequently, of the escape of worms into the stomach and even out of the body by way of the mouth or anus.

Strongyloides

Very small, slender worms, *Strongyloides westeri*, occur in the small intestine of nursing foals and are believed to be responsible, at least in part, for the high incidence of scouring among these young animals. Mature horses and mules seldom harbor this species.

The parasitic adults live in intimate contact with the lining of the gut and reproduce asexually. Eggs are liberated into the lumen and have already developed embryos when they pass out with the feces. These are usually the first parasite eggs to appear in the feces of young foals. The larvae hatch in a day or so and are capable of undergoing alternative cycles of development, either transforming directly into infective larvae or growing into free-living, bisexual adults. The latter mate in the manure or on the ground, and the females lay eggs which, in turn, develop into larvae that are infective to equines. The entire cycle is completed within a few days. It is not known whether horses acquire infection by direct skin penetration by the larvae, although this is probable, or by ingesting the larvae during grazing or in contaminated water. At post mortem inspection, the presence of *Strongyloides* may be suspected if the mucous membrane of the upper part of the small intestine exhibits localized inflammation and reddening. The worms can be removed by scraping, and a diagnosis can be made with a low-power microscope.

Pinworms

Whitish worms with long slender tails, pinworms (*Oxyuris equi*) are frequently seen in the feces of heavily infected animals. This fact at once suggests a useful method of diagnosing pinworm infection and an important point in the developmental cycle of this parasite. The worms mature in the large intestine, principally in the dorsal colon, the females becoming full of eggs as they proceed along the small colon toward the rectum. Sometimes the females crawl out of the anal opening and then rupture, leaving the eggs glued to the perianal region. The resultant irritation and itching cause their affected animal to rub itself against posts or other objects, and this frequently leads to secondary infection, which accentuates the discomfort. Rubbing may also crush more female worms on the perianal surfaces. Normally, however, the eggs develop on the ground or in manure and infection is acquired as in the case of the large roundworms.

Male pinworms are much smaller than the females and appear to live principally in the dorsal colon. In this region also are found at post mortem examination many fourth-stage larvae, which are peculiarly equipped with large muscular mouths for attachment to the mucosa and for voracious feeding.

In addition to the perianal injury produced by pinworms, there is the possibility that the eggs or the matrix of the uterine substance in which they are embedded may have some peculiarly irritating property. The fourth-stage larvae are also injurious on account of their mode of life within the colon. Diagnosis can be made by finding the characteristic eggs in perianal scrapings or by the discovery of adult worms in the manure. Tail rubbing is presumptive evidence of infection.

Pinworms of another species, *Probstmayria vivipara*, are frequently present in large numbers in equines, but they are so small as to be scarcly visible to the unaided eye. These are viviparous worms, as their species name implies–that is, the young are born alive, the eggs being hatched within the body of the female–and they can presumable complete their entire cycle of development in the ventral colon of the host. Nothing is known of the injuriousness of this species or of its means of transmission from horse to horse.

Lungworms

Lungworms of the species *Dictyocaulus arnfieldi*, which live in the bronchi and bronchioles of horses, are of scattered occurrence in the United States and elsewhere. In heavy infections they cause a chronic cough and bronchitis, which weaken the host animal.

The females produce eggs with embryos which hatch in the lungs soon after deposition. The embryos are coughed up through the trachea or are carried up by the action of its ciliated lining. Then, in general, they are swallowed and pass out through the alimentary tract, though in some cases they are expelled from the body during coughing or sneezing. The larvae become infective within a week or so and produce infections in new hosts that swallow them. Larvae reach the lungs after a migration somewhat similar to that of the large roundworms and grow to maturity there.

Filariae

Of the several species of filariae which have been described as being found in equines, many are known only by their larval stages (micro-filariae) and it is probable that some, at least, are identical. Only two are of common occurrence.

One of these, *Setaria equina*, is the well-known threadworm of the abdominal cavity. It lives normally in intimate association with the supporting tissues of the intestine, but it is sufficiently large (about 4 inches long) and active to be easily detected at post mortem examination. So far as is known, this parasite does hot usually produce serious injury. Infections consisting of a dozen or more threadworms are however, capable of causing inflammation of the lining of the body cavity and effusion of fluid into this region; 10 liters (about 2½ gallons) or more of free fluid may be present in the abdominal cavity as a result. Occasionally, also, the immature forms of this filaria get into the eyes and cause severe disturbance and serious local injury.

The other filarial worm, *Onchoceroa reticulata*, parasitizes the ligamentum nuchae (the large tendon supporting the neck) and is believed to have an important role in the development of poll evil and fistulous withers. Not infrequently, infection with this species leaves only chalklike, elongate nodules or bundles buried in the ligamentous tissue. Recent studies suggest that the microfilariae of this parasite are responsible for skin lesions in horses and probably for the condition referred to as dhobie itch.

Both of the species named have indirect life cycles, horses probably acquiring infection from the bites of infected insect hosts. Although the vectors of *Setaria equina* have not been definitely determined. It has been shown by recent studies that *Onchocerca reticulata* is transmitted by tiny biting flies known as midges.

Treatment for Protozoan Diseases

Two kinds of agents are used with some success in the treatment of the trypanosome diseases of equines–antimony compounds and synthetic metal-free organic chemicals. The antimony compound first used successfully is tartar emetic (antimony potassium tartrate).

Though very effective, this is also very toxic. It is administered by injection into the veins and care must be taken that no trace of the drug gets into the tissues. With colts and shy animals that jump at the prick of the needle, it is difficult to prevent the escape of the drug into surrounding tissue. This will cause swelling and abscess formation and, in the more severe cases, a sloughing of tissue about the site of injection. Principally to avoid these objectionable effects, many other antimony compounds have been tested against the equine tryponosomes. From the evidence available it is impossible to select the most valuable of these substances but a proprietary drug manufactured and sold under the name "Fuadin."[3] may be taken as an example of the advantages and disadvantages that have accrued from this type of investigation. This compound may be given by either intravenous or intramuscular injection, and it is less acutely toxic than tartar emetic. Apparently, however, animals treated with this drug are more likely to relapse than are those treated with tartar emetic. Also Fuadin is the more expensive of the two and is considered uneconomical for use in some localities.

Several arsenicals have also been tested. Arsenic is a metal very similar chemically to antimony. Although some investigators have reported successful results with one or another of the arsenic compounds, the reports suggest that in general they are less effective than are the antimony compounds.

The only synthetic, metal-free, organic compound that has been used extensively and successfully in equine trypanosomiasis is a complex urea derivative.[4] The drug is dissolved in water and injected either intravenously or intramuscularly. Usually the treatment is repeated after a fortnight. The trypanosomes in the peripheral (exterior) circulation are quickly destroyed, and sometimes a complete cure is obtained. Many relapses, however, have followed this treatment, though some of these, and possibly all, may have been caused by organisms that had invaded the spinal fluid prior to treatment or by failure to administer a curative dose of the drug. Some investigators have injected this as well as other drugs directly

---

[3] A 6.7 percent sclution of sodium-antimony III bis-pyrocatechin disulfonate of sodium having a pH of 7, and containing 13.5 percent of trivalent antimony.

[4] This is marketed under many names but is best known as Bayer 205, Germanin, and Naganol.

into the neural canal (in the backbone), which is often a reservoir of infection. Some successes have been reported with this technique, but the method is not practicable on a large scale. In brief, then, this drug may be employed most effectively in early infections but is of limited value in the more advanced cases.

After extensive experience with murrina in Panama, investigators there resorted to a combination of the drug mentioned above with one of the metallic compounds. The intravenous injection of a solution containing 1.3 grams (21 grains) of tartar emetic and 0.5 gram (8 grains) of Bayer 205 has given good results in many cases, but the frequency of relapses makes it impossible to recommend this as a wholly satisfactory method of treatment.

Because of its powerful action in killing trypanosomes, Bayer 205 has been used as a disease preventive with some success. Injections of the drug at triweekly intervals have been found to provide satisfactory protection against infection, but the expense of this procedure is often prohibitive. Moreover, many animals react unfavorably to repeated administrations of this drug.

Many remedies have been tried for piroplasmosis. The most satisfactory seems to be a compound known as acaprin or akiron.[5] It is given either subcutaneously (under the skin) or intramuscularly, and in many cases a single injection is sufficient. In some animals it has caused undesirable side reactions, which, however, are reported to have been avoided to a large extent when the drug was administered in conjunction with a substance known as rephrin. Formerly a proprietary remedy (akiron R) was manufactured that contained rephrin as well as acaprin.

Treatment for Parasitic Worms

For stomach worms (*Habrronema* species, and others) and large roundworms (*Parascaris equorum*), carbon disulfide is the most commonly used anthelmintic. The chemical is given to animals after they have fasted 18 hours and is administered in doses of about 6 fluid drams. Ordinarily the drug should be given by stomach tube, but a skillful veterinarian may be able to administer it satisfactorily in capsules. Carbon disulfide is irritating to the membranes of the mouth, and for this reason it must be carefully administered to avoid

[5] Chemically, N, N[1]- (Bismethyl-chinolylium-methylsulfate-6).

contact with them. It also causes marked inflammation of the membranes of the stomach and occasionally produces other unfavorable reactions. The latter are sometimes counteracted by a purgative dose of magnesium sulfate, administered some time after the anthelmintic.

The large numbers and wide distribution of strongyles have given rise to the use and development of many anthelmintics for their removal. Most of these remove only part of the worms, whereas others which are effective cause more or less severe intoxication, or poisoning. The traditional drug used against these parasites is oil of chenopodium. It is very effective and quite safe, but animals are usually slow to recover from the after effects. Carbon tetrachloride is also effective but has proved toxic under certain conditions. Normal butylidene chloride, although effective, has never been widely used because of its high cost. A closely related chemical, normal butylidene chloride, which seems to be equally effective, is less expensive but is unfortunately metabolized in the horse to a very unpleasant smelling substance. All these drugs must be given after an extended fast and must be followed by a purgative.

Workers in the Federal Bureau of Animal Industry have recently introduced a new anthelmintic, phenothiazine, which seems to lack most of the objectionable features of the drugs previously used. It should be given without a preliminary fast and need not be followed by a purgative. This new drug is highly effective for the removal of strongyles, and it is usually nontoxic in therapeutic doses, although a temporary anemia and some jaundice frequently follow its administration. An occasional death is reported to have been caused by phenothiazine, although thousands of horses have been successfully treated. Its contraindications (conditions under which the drug cannot be used safely) and incompatibilities are incompletely determined, but present evidence indicates that the advantages of phenothiazine may far outweigh any disadvantages that might accompany its use. The therapeutic dose is 30 to 50 grams (1 to 1¾ ounces) for an adult equine. It may be administered by capsule, by stomach tube, or by mixing the drug with suitable feedstuffs. It is important that doses be prepared separately for each animal and that animals be dosed individually. Phenothiazine may be made into a satisfactory suspension for use as a drench by mixing one dose of the drug with 20 cubic centimeters (two-thirds ounce) of molasses and adding enough water to make 90 cubic centimeters (3 fluid ounces). In order to obtain a smooth mixture, the water must be added in small quantities and stirred into the molasses-phenothiazine mixture after each addition of the fluid. When medicated feed mixtures are used, the drug may be mixed with almost any suitable ground feed or mixed gram. It is simplest merely to moisten the feed (2 to 2½ quarts of feed to one dose) and mix in the drug. If this medicated mixture is fed in lieu of a regular afternoon feeding, horses will usually consume it during the night.

Control Measures

Since most equine parasites owe their perpetuation to the fact that the animals graze or take their feed from the same places that they deposit their feces, a good deal can be accomplished toward reducing parasitism and keeping animals in good condition by providing sanitary stables and good pastures and by avoiding overstocking. Manure should be removed frequently from stables, which should be of good construction and kept clean. Before spreading the manure out as fertilizer, it is important, if practicable, to destroy the parasite eggs and larvae contained in it. Eggs and larvae are killed by spontaneously generated heat if the manure is stored in a specially constructed, insulated box for 2 or 3 weeks before being used. Grain boxes and hay racks should be so placed as to avoid contamination with manure. Attention to these details and periodic medication for worms are the best general measures for keeping horses free from parasites.

Chapter 8

MANGE IN EQUINES

Marion Imes[1]

[1] *Marion Imes is Senior Veterinarian, Zoological Division, Bureau of Animal Industry.*

Nature, it seems, has ingeniously devised, for each kind of livestock, a set of mites that live at the expense of the host animals and their owners. Here is an account of the creatures that make horses mangy, and how to get rid of these tormenting pests.

Mange in equines, also known as scabies, scab, or itch, includes a group of contagious skin diseases affecting horses, asses, and mules. Since for practical purposes the causes, symptoms, diagnosis, and treatment of mange in the three kinds of animals are similar, mange in horses is selected as typical of the disease in the group.

Mange is caused by small insect like parasites known as mites which live on or in the skin of the host animal. Horses are commonly infected by three different genera of mange mites–*Sarcoptes, Psoroptes,* and *Chorioptes*-and each causes a different kind of mange, known as sarcoptic, psoroptic, and chorioptic, respectively.

Mange mites are truly parasitic, as their entire life cycles are passed on the host animal, and they are the sole cause of mange in equines. In obtaining their food from the tissues of the host and carrying on other life processes, the mites cause wounds or lesions in the skin. As each class of mites has distinctive habits, the nature and location of the lesions they cause in the early stages of mange are sufficiently characteristic to aid in making a differential diagnosis–that is, a diagnosis of the specific type of mange in a given case.

Contagiousness of Mange

Each species of domesticated animal has its own peculiar varieties of mange mites, and most of the mites from one species of animal cannot live and propagate permanently on a different species. The sarcoptic mites, however, are transmissible from one species of animal to another and some, including the sarcoptic mites of the horse from animals to man. Ordinarily when one species of animal contracts the contagion from another species, the mites live only a limited time on the new host.

Mange is usually transmitted by direct contact with infected animals, but equipment used on or around infected animals or other objects in contact with them act as carriers from which the disease may be contracted. Although mange mites cannot complete their life cycles off the host animal, they may live as long as 2 months when dislodged in cool moist places, and the eggs may retain their vitality for about 4 weeks. Since various factors such as exposure to sunlight, dry air, and other conditions affect the longevity of mites and the viability of their eggs when separated from their host, it is not known definitely how long infected premises may remain a source of danger. Practical experience indicates that buildings and corrals are free from infection about 30 days after all infected animals have been removed.

The spread of mange from one animal to another is not limited to anyone season of the year, although the mites are usually most active on the host animals during the winter months. The disease spreads rapidly among horses closely confined or crowded together. Animals exposed to sunlight on pasture seldom contract mange or show new lesions. If they are infected, however, the disease will become active under winter conditions.

Mange is very contagious to horses of all ages and classes, and precautions should be taken to prevent the introduction, spread, or harboring of the contagion. Untreated infected animals or objects used on or around such animals should not come in contact with horses free from the disease. If the disease occurs, all horses on, the premises should be treated regardless of the number showing, infection. All buildings and small inclosures occupied by infected horses and all equipment used in or around such horses, should be cleaned and disinfected. All litter should be removed from buildings and yards and the exposed surfaces should be sprayed with coal-tar-creosote dip or disinfectant (see Disinfection and Disinfectants), diluted in accordance with the instructions on the container. Equipment which may carry the mites should be immersed in the disinfectant.

Sarcoptic Mange

The minute white or yellowish parasites that cause sarcoptic, or common, mange of horses are known technically as *Sarcoptes scabiei equi.* The full-grown female mite is about one-fiftieth of an inch and the male about one-sixtieth of an inch in length. They are barely visible to the naked eye but are plainly visible under an ordinary hand lens. The general form of the body is more nearly round than oval, and under a high-power microscope a number of short spines projecting backward may be seen on its upper surface. When mature, these mites have four pairs of short thick legs. The first and second pairs near the head extend beyond the margin of the body, but the third and fourth pairs usually are not visible unless the mite is placed on its back or dorsal surface.

The sarcoptic mites penetrate the upper layer of skin and form burrows or galleries in which mating occurs and the eggs are laid. Each female forms a separate burrow and lays from 10 to 25 eggs. The eggs hatch in from 3 to 10 days, and the young mites after passing through several molts begin laying eggs in new burrows when they are 10 to 12 days old. The average period of incubation (from the time the eggs are laid until they hatch) is about 4 days, and the average period from hatching until egg laying begins is about 11 days. A new generation of mites, therefore, may be produced in about 15 days.

The first visible symptoms of sarcoptic mange in horses are the signs the animal manifests of an intense localized itching. The burrows formed by the mites usually extend to the sensitive layer of the skin, and the presence and activities of the parasites in the tissues cause irritation, inflammation, and swelling. Vesicles (blisters) and small nodules, or lumps, are formed in the skin over and around the burrows. The vesicles break and discharge serum which may dry into scales or granules.

The disease may start on any part of the body, but usually the first lesions appear on the neck, shoulders, or head. From these parts they spread until the entire body may become involved. As the disease advances the nodules become closer together, the hair over the lesions stands erect, and some of it drops out. The skin becomes swollen, thick, and dense to the touch and is drawn into wrinkles or folds. The mechanical injury to the skin from rubbing and biting causes large scabs to form. When the mites are not very active the skin may have a dry, leather like appearance.

The only certain method of diagnosis is to demonstrate the presence of the mite. If the lesions are moist, the mites can usually be found in scrapings taken from the edge of a fresh lesion or the furrows of the wrinkles. As sarcoptic mites live in the skin and not on the surface, it is necessary to scrape down to the second or sensitive layer of skin to obtain them. When the lesions are dry and the skin has a leatherlike appearance, it is difficult to find the mites.

Psoroptic Mange

The mites, called *Psoroptes communis equi*, which cause psoroptic mange in horses are slightly larger than sarcoptic mites. They are visible to the naked eye, especially when they are placed against a dark background. The general form of the body is oval, and the tapering head is longer than it is broad. When mature, the mites have four pairs of legs, all extending beyond the margin of the body.

The psoroptic mites do not form burrows but live in colonies on the surface of the skin. Each female may deposit as many as 24 eggs, which hatch on the animal in 4 to 7 days. The new generation of mites reach maturity and mate, and the females deposit eggs in from 10 to 12 days from the time of hatching. These stages in the life cycle have an important bearing on the interval between treatments.

Psoroptic mange is more contagious. and usually spreads more rapidly than the sarcoptic variety. The disease usually starts on those parts of the body covered thickly by hair. In obtaining their food the mites puncture the skin of the host animal and probably introduce a poisonous secretion into the wound. As the mites increase, many small wounds are made, causing intense itching, inflammation, formation of vesicles, and exudation of serum. The serum on the surface of the lesion becomes mixed with foreign matter, including micro-organisms, and the mass soon hardens into small yellowish or gray-colored scabs. As the scabs form, the mites move to and feed on the healthy skin around the edges of the lesion, and thus the scab-covered wound is gradually enlarged. The scabs may become dark-colored from blood stains and other causes.

Some of the mites move to other parts of the body and form new lesions, and the process is continued until the entire body surface may become involved. As the disease advances, increasingly large areas of skin become denuded of hair and covered with adherent crusts or scabs. The areas of affected skin become thickened and hardened, or else swollen. The severe itching causes the infected animals to rub, bite, or scratch themselves, so that the scabs are often broken and some of them are torn loose, leaving bleeding wounds. Animals with advanced cases of mange become weak and emaciated, and unless relieved by proper treatment, many of them die.

Psoroptic mites may be seen on the skin, but to demonstrate the presence of the mites it is usually necessary to scrape the outer edges of a red moist lesion with a dull knife blade and transfer the scrapings to a smooth black surface, such as a piece of black paper or a painted board. Spreading the scrapings in the warm sum or near artificial heat usually causes the mites to become active, and they can be seen as minute, gray, moving bodies against the dark background. They are quite plainly visible under a low-power hand lens.

Chorioptic Mange

Chorioptic mange, commonly known as foot or tail mange, is a contagious skin disease caused by mites called *Chorioptes equi*, which closely resemble those of the psoroptic species. The chorioptic mites live on the surface of the skin and cause lesions similar to those of psoroptic mange. One characteristic difference is the location of the lesions, which are usually confined to the lower parts of the limbs or tail, though they may spread over the legs and even the abdomen.

For practical purposes it is not necessary to differentiate between chorioptic and psoroptic mange, as the treatment is the same for both diseases. If the lesions are confined to the lower parts of the limbs, wading tanks instead of dipping vats may be used in treatment.

Treatment of Mange

In treating horses, asses, and mules for mange the primary purpose is to kill the parasites that cause the disease. As mange mites may be on any or all parts of the skin of infected animals, eradication usually can be effected only by applying medication over the entire surface of the skin. Hand application of suitable remedies delays the spread of mange, but on account of the difficulty of applying treatment by hand over the entire body surface, the method cannot be depended upon to eradicate the disease. Hand applications are of value, however, in connection with spraying or dipping. Lesions that are covered by hard scabs or crusts should be well soaked by hand with warm dip just before the animals are dipped or sprayed.

Dipping, which consists in immersing animals in a medicated liquid that will kill mange mites, is the most effective and dependable method of treating equines for mange. A dipping vat with attached draining pens, corrals, and other necessary structures is commonly called a dipping plant, Dipping plants are usually so arranged that animals enter one end of a vat filled with dip, swim through the liquid, and leave the vat at the opposite end. Cattle-dipping plants[2] are suitable for dipping horses.

In dipping horses the depth of the liquid in the vat is usually maintained at from 70 to 80 inches, or deep enough to swim the tallest animal. Horses carry out of the vat and retain from 2 to 4 quarts of dip each, depending on their size and the condition of their hair. The total estimated quantity to be carried out by the animals to be dipped, plus that required to charge the vat, should equal the total quantity required to complete the dipping if none is lost by leakage or otherwise wasted.

The capacity of the vat is usually obtained by multiplying the average length in inches by the average width, and then multiplying the product by the depth from the dip line to the bottom, measured at the center of the vat. This gives approximately the number of cubic

---

[2] IMES, MARION. CATTLE SCAB AND METHODS OF CONTROL AND ERADICATION, U.S. Dept. Agr. Farmers' Bul. 1017, 29 pp., illus. 1918.

inches of space to be filled with dip. Divide this by 231 (the number of cubic inches in a gallon) and the result will be the number of gallons of dip needed to charge the vat. To obtain the average length and width of a vat with sloping sides, add the measurement at the bottom to that at the dip line and divide by 2.

After the vat is charged, the contents should be well stirred so that the dip may be of uniform strength and temperature throughout. While the animals are in the vat, the head of each one should be submerged or ducked twice for an instant, and if the inner surfaces of the ears are not well soaked they should be hand-treated, Mangy horses are usually held in the dip for 2 to 3 minutes.

When only a few horses are to be treated and a dipping vat is not available, the dip can be applied in the form of a spray. This method is not economical but if the spraying is continued until the entire surface of the skin is well soaked, mange can be eradicated in this way, An orchard spraying outfit or an ordinary hand spray pump is suitable for the purpose.

Two dippings 10 to 12 days apart usually effect eradication of psoroptic and chorioptic mange. The first dipping, if properly done, kills all the mites but does not destroy the eggs. The second dipping, if timed correctly, kills the new generation of mites before they start laying eggs.

Sarcoptic mites are more difficult to eradicate. One dipping usually does not kill all the mites, probably because the dip does not always reach the bottom of all their burrows and come in contact with all them. The proper interval between dippings for sarcoptic mange is 6 or 7 days, and four or more dippings or treatments are usually necessary to eradicate the disease in ordinary cases. Old chronic cases which have continued for several years are practically incurable, and animals so infested should be isolated or slaughtered.

Two classes of dips commonly and successfully used are lime-sulfur and nicotine. Both are used warm for dipping horses; the temperature of the dip in the vat is usually maintained at 90° to 95° F. while in use. Prepared dips should be diluted or mixed and used in accordance with the instructions on the label of the container.

Proprietary brands of lime-sulfur are available either as a concentrated liquid, known as liquid lime-sulfur, or as powder or crystals, known as dry lime-sulfur. These products are equal to or even better than the home-made lime-sulfur dip.[3]

The nicotine dips sold under various trade names are effective remedies for mange when diluted with water so that the dip contains not less than 0.05 percent nicotine. If used much stronger, they are likely to injure horses, especially if the animals are warm from exercise or hot weather, or if very hard water is used in diluting the dip. Nicotine dips should not be heated above 110° F.

[3] SCHWARZ, BENJAMIN, IMES, MARION, and WRIGHT, WILLARD H. PARASITES AND PARASITIC DISEASES OF HORSES. U.S. Dept. Agr. Cir. 148, 54 pp., illus. 1930.

Chapter 9

HORSE BOTS AND THEIR CONTROL

F.C. Bishopp & Benjamin Schwartz[1]

[1] *F.C. Bishopp is Assistant Chief, Bureau of Entomology and Plant Quarantine and Benjamin Schwartz is Principle Zoologist and Chief of the Zoological Division, Bureau of Animal Industry.*

For sheer inventiveness in accomplishing their objects, it would be hard to beat the insects, and it would seem that the devil himself must have invented the methods used by botflies to reach the viscera of horses. Fortunately, man has brains that can be pitted with reasonable success against instinct.

Horse bots are highly specialized parasites that attack horses, mules, asses, and perhaps zebras. Bots do not molest cattle, sheep, or other, farm animals, even though they may be grazing in the same pasture with horses. If the horses are removed from such a pasture, the botflies will die without laying their eggs on the other animals.

Occasionally a young horse bot is found in the skin of a human being, who is evidently an accidental and unfavorable host. Under these conditions the bots act very differently from the way they do in horses; they burrow rapidly about in the skin and have never been known to grow to any considerable size or to reach the stomach or intestines, where they normally attach themselves in horses. In the human skin the minute larvae cause severe itching and local irritation. The burrows may traverse the skin for several inches, leaving a raised, reddened, circuitous streak, suggesting in miniature the work of a meadow mole in a field. How the larvae get into human skin is not known, and the cases are rare.

Four distinct species of bots have been found in the United States, but one of them is extremely rare. The other three are serious pests of horses and mules. They are known as the common horse bot, or nit fly (*Gastrophilus intestinalis*); the throat bot, or chin fly (*G. nasalis*); and the nose bot, or nose fly (*G. haemorrhoidalis*).[2]

Distribution

Horse bots were undoubtedly brought to this country with horses imported from Europe.

The common horse botfly and the throat botfly occur throughout the United States wherever horses are found, but they are much more numerous in some localities than in others. Throat botflies are extremely abundant in the drier parts of the country and at the higher altitudes–that is, above 3,000 feet. The presence of large numbers of horses in which they may develop favors an abundance of horse bots.

The throat bot appears to have become established in the United States comparatively recently–that is, about 1898. It was first observed in the western part of the Dakotas and in eastern Montana and since that time has spread over much of the region from Illinois to eastern Washington and Oregon, and from southern Canada to central Kansas.

With the free movement of horses and mules from infested areas to various parts of the country, it is surprising that the throat boat has not become more widespread. It is likely that climatic conditions, especially in the eastern and southern States, are not favorable for this species, and this is also probably the reason why the fourth species, the European horse bot (*G. inermis*), has not became established in the United States.

---

2 Further information on the distribution, habits, and methods of controlling bots will be found in publications by Bishopp and Dove (*1*),[3] by Dove (*4*), and by Wells and Knipling (*11*).

3 Italic numbers in parentheses refer to Literature Cited.

Losses Causes by Horse Bots

Horse owners soon become aware of the presence of horse bots because of the annoyance the flies cause the animals. This is particularly true of the nose botfly, which lays its eggs around the lips of horses. The animal attacked reacts violently. It may toss its head in the air, strike the ground with its front feet, and rub its nose on the ground, the neck yoke, or a barbed-wire fence. If a very nervous animal in harness is attacked, it may run away, and sometimes serious damage results. These flies prevent horses on pasture from grazing. The animals usually stand in groups., preferably on the highest spot available, with the nose of one resting on the back of another, as shown in Figure 1. Horses are often seen walking or trotting across a pasture with their heads constantly nodding to avoid the attacks of nose flies.

The throat botfly is also very annoying to animals when laying eggs, but less so than the nose fly. The animals become excited when attacked and often throw their heads violently upward. The common

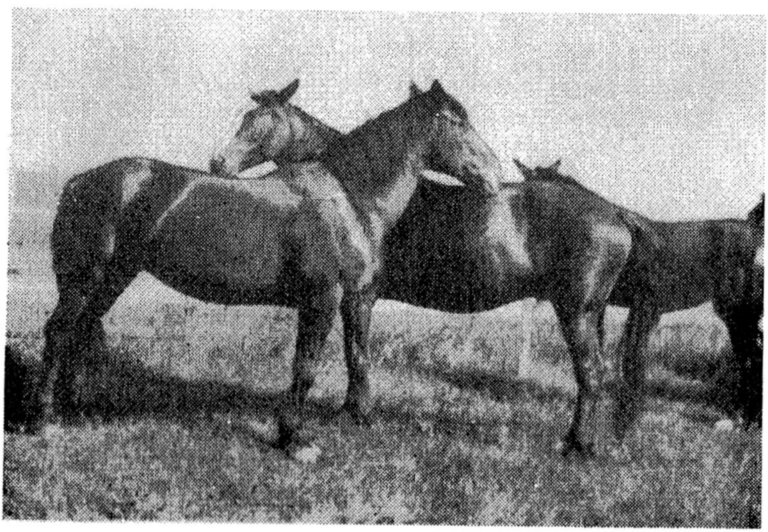

Fig. 1: Horses attempt to protect themselves from nose botflies by resting their muzzles on each other's backs.

horse botfly is much less disturbing than the other two, although nervous animals are considerably annoyed by it.

Contrary to the belief of many persons, these flies do not sting or otherwise hurt an animal. They undoubtedly cause a tickling sensation when they touch the hairs to lay their eggs, and this is probably very disturbing when the nose fly touches the edges of the lips.

The newly hatched nose bots burrow into the lips and travel around in the mucous lining of the horse's mouth; the young common bots burrow in the tongue; the first-stage throat bots infest the gums. This burrowing habit, first recorded by Dinulescu (3) in 1932, causes considerable irritation and perhaps at times interferes with feeding. En route to the stomach, the bots sometimes attach themselves in the pharynx and have been known to cause swelling of the throat sufficient to prevent the passage of food.

In the stomach and intestines, the bots remain attached for several months. At the points of attachment deep pits are formed in the lining membranes (Fig. 2), which may serve as places of entry for germs. If the infestation is very heavy, digestion may be seriously interfered with, and clusters of bots attached at the exited of the stomach may impede the passage of food. These conditions give rise to colic, lowered vitality, and reduced work output. The nose bot has the habit also of reattaching itself in the rectum as it passes out, and there again it causes irritation and itching.

Much of the damage caused by bots in the mouth and digestive tract of horses is not recognized by stock owners, but it is none the less important and causes farmers heavy losses.

Life History and Habits

Like other flies, horse bots pass through four distinct stages– the egg, the larva (bot), the pupa, and the adult. The adult botflies are unable to take food; enough is stored up in their bodies in the bot stage to develop the 150 to 300 eggs to be deposited during the short life of the adult fly, whose sole purpose is reproduction. During favorable weather many eggs are laid in a short time.

In 1938 Wells and Knipling (*11*) presented information on the habits and life histories of these common species.

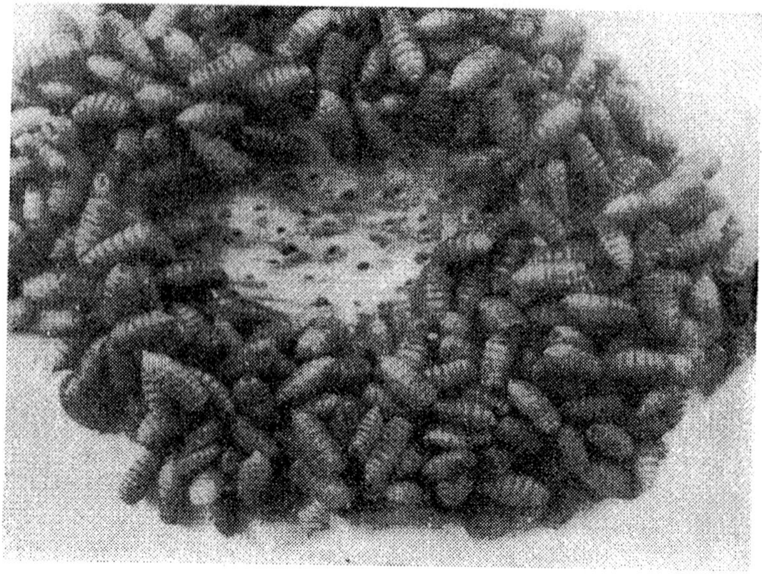

Fig. 2: Some of the bots from a horse's stomach, with a section of the stomach lining in the center showing pits made by bots.

The eggs of all the species are attached to hairs of the host, but there is considerable difference in the place of attachment and also in the shape and color of the eggs (Fig. 3). The common botfly lays its eggs on various parts of the animal, but particularly on the inside of the knees; the throat botfly attaches its eggs toward the base of the hairs beneath the jaws; and the nose botfly deposits its eggs on the short hairs on the lips. The egg of the last species has a stalk on the base that extends well down into the hair follicle.

The egg-laying habits of the three species of botflies prevalent in this country are also different. The common botfly hovers around the legs of the horse with its abdomen curved under, depositing egg after egg. It is a large fly resembling a bee, with the wings conspicuosly spotted (Fig. 4). The other two species have plain, clear wings, are slightly smaller and darker in color, and fly more rapidly. In depositing eggs they usually approach quickly, hover beneath the

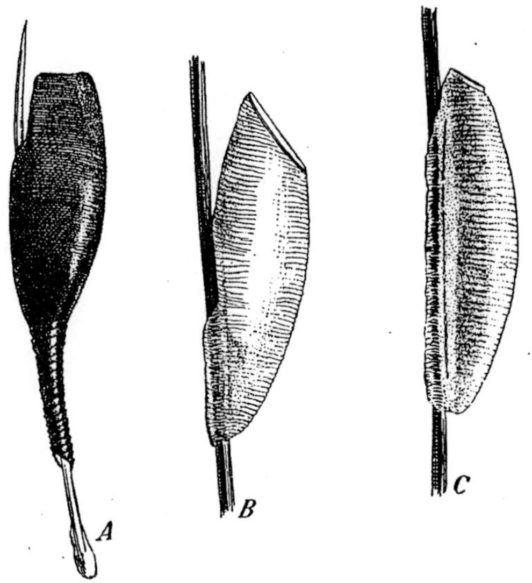

Fig. 3: Eggs of horse bots, each attached to a horsehair. A: Nose bot egg–hair removed with root; B: common horse bot egg; C: throat bot egg. Greatly enlarged.

head for an instant, and then suddenly dart at the lips or at some spot beneath the jaws, according to the species. Usually only a single egg is laid at each strike.

The eggs of the throat botfly hatch in about 6 days, and the young bots immediately crawl into the horse's mouth. Schroeder (*9*) has shown that they soon establish themselves in pockets between the molar teeth, where they grow and molt to the second stage. After 3 to 4 weeks in the mouth they pass to the stomach and intestine, where they attach themselves in the pyloric, or exit, end of the stomach and in the duodenum just below the stomach.

The eggs of the nose botfly hatch in 2 to 4 days, and the minute, spiny larvae penetrate the skin of the horse's lips and work toward the mucous lining, where they continue to burrow for more than a month before passing to the stomach.

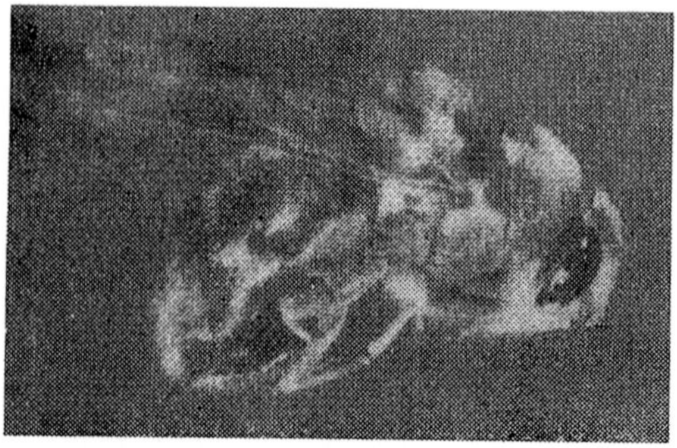

Fig. 4: Common horse botfly, or nit fly.

The eggs of the common botfly are ready to hatch 7 days after being laid on the horse's legs, but hatching does not take place until they are rubbed by the warm lips of the horse. The bots may lie quietly in the eggs as long as 3 months awaiting this stimulus. When the horse bites the spot where the eggs are embedded, it warms them, and the bots push off the egg cap and adhere to the animal's moist lips. They soon penetrate the mucous covering of the lips and tongue. Wehr *(10)* found that they burrow there for about a month before going to the stomach. During this time they molt, or cast their skins, and increase considerably in size.

All three species of bots remain attached to the lining of the digestive tract for 8 to 11 months, during which time they grow to robust tough-skinned bots about three-quarters of an inch in length. The young bots are distinctly reddish, which may indicate that they feed on blood. When mature, the throat bots are a dirty white and the common bots and nose bots pinkish. The bots of the last species take on a distinctly greenish color just before leaving the animal. When grown, the bots release their hold and pass out with the excrement, except that the nose bots reattach themselves in the rectum for a few days before dropping to the ground. They are often seen attached to the edge of the anus, from which they protrude.

The mature bots differ somewhat in size as well as color, and the species are easily distinguished by differences in their spiny armature (Fig. 5).

When the bots reach the ground they seek any protection at hand, or they may burrow just beneath the surface of the soil. In 1 to 4 days the outer skin of the bot contracts and hardens, forming a protecting case in which the change from the sluggish, repulsive maggot to an active, ornate fly takes place. The duration of the pupal, or resting, stage is similar in each species and lasts from 20 to 70 days, depending on the temperature.

In general, botflies are most abundant in late summer and fall, although in the North Central States they may begin activity about the middle of June. In southwestern Texas, the common botfly has a period of activity in the spring that ends when hot dry summer weather sets in; the flies appear again in the fall. Botfly activity ceases with the advent of freezing weather. In the warmer parts of Texas it may extend well into December.

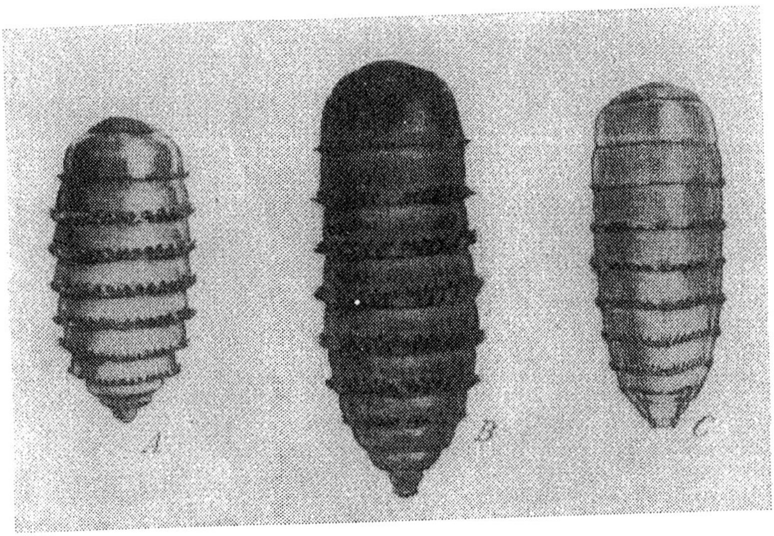

Fig. 5: The three species of bots, when full-grown, can be distinguished by their size, color, and the arrangement of spines on their bodies: A: Nose hot; B: common bot; C: throat bot.

Protecting Horses Against Botflies

Since botflies do not feed, there is no way of attracting them to traps or poisoned baits. Animals are given little protection by the use of repellents, and nets and fringes also are of little value.

As the throat botfly deposits its eggs beneath the jaws and the nose botfly on the lips, covering those areas when the flies are active largely prevents infestation and also greatly relieves animals from annoyance by the flies. It is difficult to provide such protection for animals on pasture, although protective devices have been used even there. While animals are in harness, the throat botfly can be largely warded off by placing a piece of burlap beneath the jaws with one end attached to the throatlatch and the other to the bit rings.

Various types of protectors against the nose botfly are in use. One of the simplest and best is a piece of belting, or even of an old automobile-tire, casing, 4 to 6 inches wide. This is attached at each end by a string or by snaps (Fig. 6). The protector should not be drawn tightly against the mouth, and it should be long enough to cover the lips entirely, including the corners.

The incubation period, especially that of the throat bot and the nose fly, is so short that control by destruction of the eggs is impractical because of the frequency with which an ovicide would have to be applied. Moreover, no effective egg-destroying agent has been found for these two species.

The incubation period of the common horse bot is longer, but the eggs are very resistant to destruction. Kerosene oil and creosote dips often recommended as washes for the destruction of the eggs or nits of this species, are of little value. However, a simple and effective method of destroying the eggs in the fall was discovered by Wells and Knipling (*11*). It consists of applying water at a temperature of 105° to 110° F. with a sponge or swab. Applying the warm water with vigorous rubbing causes a high percentage of the eggs to hatch and the larvae quickly die.

Treatment for the Removal of Bots

Of the remedies that have been proposed from time to time for the removal of botfly larvae from the stomach and upper part of the intestines of horses and mules, only carbon bisulfide has withstood

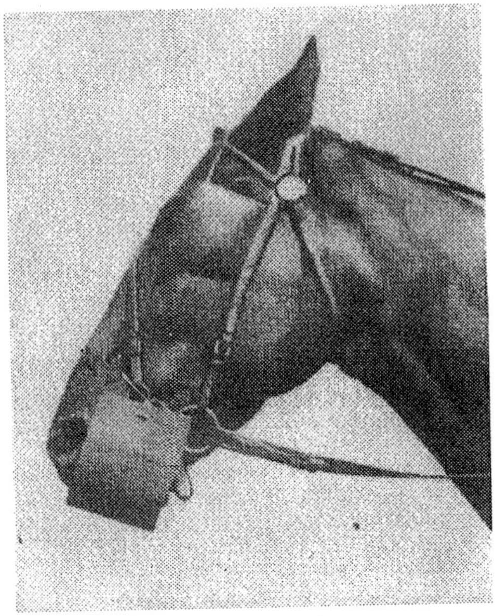

Fig. 6: A piece of belting attached to the bit rings is the best protector against nose botfly attack.

the test of rigid, critical, and painstaking experimentation (5, 6, 7, 8). A 6-dram dose, administered by stomach tube or in gelatin capsules, has become the standard treatment for a horse weighing about 1,000 pounds. For horses of other weights the dose is computed on the basis of 1.5 fluid drams (6 cubic centimeters) for each 250 pounds of weight.

This treatment should be administered not earlier than 1 month rafter the first killing frost, following a fast of 18 hours, and no purgative should be given. Although carbon bisulfide is a toxic substance, it is quite safe for horses provided it is given with due caution by a competent veterinarian. The volatile liquid produces a limited area of inflammation in the stomach of a horse or mule, but this is not known to have serious consequences and disappears in a week or two. When the capsule is administered by inexperienced persons, however, there is danger that it may break in the mouth, with alarming and possibly dangerous consequences. This treatment destroys practically all of the bots in the digestive tract, and also many of the large roundworms that may be there.

Mass or solid capsules containing carbon bisulfide adsorbed on magnesium carbonate came into vogue a number of years ago as a substitute for the liquid carbon bisulfide. Critical tests by Bozicevich and Underwood (2) on seven horses showed that the solid capsule was not nearly so dependable as the liquid drug. These investigators also observed that the solid capsules became brittle with age and finally cracked and that over a period of several months they diminished in weight, owing to the decomposition of the carbon bisulfide and the escape of hydrogen sulfide. The liquid drug, then, is considered the best preparation to use for the removal of bots from horses and mules. When carbon bisulfide as put up by veterinary supply houses in gelatin capsules in administered, care should be taken to see that the capsules are still flexible. If they are brittle they should not be used.

Time of Year for Treatment

The time of year when the treatment is given is important. In most parts of the country the greatest success is obtained by treating during December and January. In the extreme South, January is preferable. It is desirable, of course, to remove the bots early in the season in order to put the horses through the winter in the best condition possible, but to prevent reinfestation, treatment must not be given until all botfly activity has been stopped by cold weather. Hot water is then applied to all parts of the body where there are eggs of the common botfly. Thirty to forty days is then allowed to elapse to give time for the young bots to pass from the mucous membranes of the mouth to the stomach, where the carbon bisulfide can reach and kill them.

Although many bots can be destroyed by treating the horses at any time of year, if treatment is delayed until spring many of the bots may have matured and passed out, and some of the nose bots may have passed down into the lower intestine, where they are less readily reached by medication.

Community Campaigns

One of the most practical developments in medication for the removal of bots from equines is the community or area campaign for eradication by medicinal treatment of horses and mules. In the it Middle West the South, and elsewhere, these campaigns have been carried out with considerable success. As a rule, area or community treatment is supported and arranged for by the county agent or farm adviser. Under Ideal conditions, all the horses in a given area are treated at the same time and at one place or in a limited number of places where the animals are assembled. The treatment is administered by veterinarians, practically all of the veterinarians in the community participating in the work. So far as can be ascertained, there has been no dissatisfaction with this method on the part of the veterinarians administering the treatments or of the farmers engaging in such cooperative efforts. In all instances liquid carbon bisulfide in capsules is administered to the horses, which have been kept on a fast for 18 hours. Area or community treatment has great advantages over individual treatment not only because it affords professional services at a minimum price but also because it may pave the way for complete eradication of bots from horses and mules in the area.

Literature Cited

(1) BISHOPP, F.C. and DOVE, W.E. (1926). THE HORSE HOTS AND THEIR CONTROL. U.S. Dept. Agr. Farmers' Bul. 1503, 14 pp., illus.

(2) BOZICEVICH, JOHN, and UNDERWOOD, PAUL C. (1932). CRITICAL EXPERIMENTS WITH SOLID CARBON DISULPHATE CAPSULES FOR THE TREATMENT OF GASTROPHILUS SPP IN THE HORSE. Vet. Med. 27: 360-364. illus.

(3) DINULESCU, G. (1932). RECHERCHES SUR LA BIOLOGIE DES GASTROPHILES. ANATOMIE. PHYSIOLOGIE, CYCLE EVOLUTIF. Ann. des Sci. Nat., Zool., ser. X, t. XV, fasc. 1, 183 pp. illus.

(4) DOVE, W.E. (1918). SOME BIOLOGICAL AND CONTROL STUDIES OF GASTROPHILUS HAEMORRHODALIS AND OTHER BOTS OF HORSES. U.S. Dept. Agr. Bul. 597, 52 pp., ills.

(5) HALL, MAURICE C. (1917). NOTES IN REGARD TO BOTS, GASTROPHILUS SPP. Amer. Vet. Med. Assoc. Jour. (n.s. 5) 52: 177-184.

(6) ________and AVERY, LAURENCE (1919). THE USE OF CARBON BIOSULPHIDE IN INFESTATIONS WITH BOTS. Amer. Vet. Med. Assoc. Jour. (n.s. 9) 56: 265-270.

(7) ________SMEAD, MORGAN J., and WOLF, CHARLES F. (1919). STUDIES ON ANTHELMINTICS. II. THE ANTHELMINTIC AND INSECTICIDAL VALUE OF CARBON BIOSULPHIDE AGAINST GASTRO-INTESTINAL PARASITES OF THE HORSE. Amer. Vet. Med. Assoc. Jour. (n.s. 8) 55: 543-549.

(8) PERRONCITO, E. and Bosso, G. (1894). EXPERIENCES SUB LA RESISTANCE VITALE DES LARVES D'OESTRE (GASTROPHILUS EQUI). Rec. de Med. vet. (8) 1 (21): 657-665.

(9) SCHROEDER, H.O. (1940). HABITS OF THE LARVAE OF GASTROPHILUS NASALIS (L) IN THE MOUTH OF THE HORSE. Jour. Econ. Ent. 33: 382-384.

(10) WEHR, EVERETT E. (1933). OBSERVATIONS OF THE LENGTH OF TIME FIRST-STAGE LARVAE OF GASTROPHILUS INTIBTINALI8 REMAIN IN THE TONGUE OF THE HORSE. North Amer. Vet. 14 (10): 35-41.

(11) WELLS, R.W., and KNIPLING, E.F. (1938). A REPORT OF SOME RECENT STUDIES ON SPECIES OF GASTROPHILUS OCCURRING IN HORSES IN THE UNITED STATES. Iowa State Col. Jour. Sci. 12: 181-203, illus.

Chapter 10

SOME INSECT PESTS OF HORSES AND MULES

F.C. Bishopp[1]

[1] *F.C. Bishopp is Assistant Chief. Bureau of Entomology and Plant Quarantine.*

Here is condensed and practical information about several enemies of the horse and mule, including mosquitoes, sand flies (punkies), houseflies, horseflies, deer flies, buffalo gnats (blackflies), fleas, lice, and ticks. Special attention is given to control measures.

A considerable number of insects and insect relatives attack equines in addition to the horse bots, stableflies, ticks, screwworms, and mange mites discussed in other articles in this book. Some of them, such as the biting and sucking lice of horses and mules, are specific; some, like the tropical horse tick, attack other animals but prefer to feed on equines; and many others feed on various warm-blooded animals without seeming to prefer anyone kind.

A number of such pests at times become so abundant locally as to have serious effects on horses, causing poor condition, lower work output, difficulty in handling, and even death.

Mosquitoes and Sand Flies

Many kinds of mosquitoes and sand flies, or punkies, attack horses and mules. As a rule, a moderate number of these insects do not greatly annoy horses; but the presence of large numbers sometimes constitutes a serious problem especially among high-strung animals such as race horses. Difficulties due to these insects have been encountered at meets and fairs held during the late spring and early fall in cities along the south Atlantic coast.

Screening the stables gives some protection against mosquitoes. Sand files, however, readily pass through ordinary screens, and smudges and sprays are resorted to for relief from them. Painting the screens in the evening with a mixture of 1 part pyrethrum extract concentrate and 20 parts lubricating oil (S.A.E. 5), together with the use of a pyrethrum-kerosene spray in the buildings, is effectlve.[2] Pasturing the horses on high ground free from dense woods and a underbrush reduces the mosquito and sand fly hazards outdoors.

Eliminating stagnant water in and near pastures, emptying and cleaning water troughs frequently, and, in salt marsh areas, ditching the parts of the marsh known to produce mosquitoes are effective steps in preventing trouble. Since there are many species of mosquitoes and they have widely divergent habits, control measures must be modified to fit the situation. After stagnant water has been eliminated as far as practicable, the principal lines of attack are:

(1) Apply No.2 fuel oil lightly to the surface pools where mosquito wigglers are found;

(2) Keep livestock on high, open pastures when mosquitoes are abundant;

(3) Keep valuable animals in screened barns;

(4) Use kerosene-pyrethrum sprays to kill the mosquitoes on animals and in the barns; and

(5) Make smudges in which stock may find protection during severe mosquito outbreaks.

In this brief account it is not possible to discuss all the different methods of controlling mosquitoes. The reader is therefore referred to other published articles that supply more details (*1, 4, 7*).[3]

---

[2] UNITED STATES BUREAU OF ENTOMOLOGY AND PLANT QUARANTINE. SAND FLIES AND PUNKIES. U.S. Bur. Ent. and Plant Quar. Cir. E-441, 3 pp. 1938. [Processed.]

[3] Italic numbers in parentheses refer to Literature Cited.

The fact should not be lost sight of that at least eight American species of mosquitoes have been shown to be capable of carrying equine encephalomyelitis. Epizootics, or severe outbreaks, of this disease are usually concurrent with mosquito outbreaks, and protecting animals from mosquito attack appears to be of some value in preventing the disease.

The Housefly

The housefly is not of great importance as an enemy of the horse, but, if not controlled, it breeds in tremendous numbers in horse manure. The presence of this insect in abundance is a serious hazard to human health.

The housefly annoys horses by its persistent efforts to feed on body secretions, particularly those of the eyes. This leads to the suspicion that the flies may transmit certain infectious eye diseases. The housefly is an intermediate host and transmitter of the roundworm parasite of equines, *Habronema muscae* (*8*), and it has also been shown to be capable of transmitting mastitis of cattle.

The control of houseflies depends on the proper disposal of manure and vegetable refuse (*5*). Scattering such materials thinly over fields soon to be plowed is the most satisfactory method of handing them. Manure may be stored in fly-tight manure pits or on racks over water. Treating manure with borax at the rate of 11 ounces to each 8 bushels also checks fly breeding. If the manure is to used as a fertilizer, borax should not be used in excess of this amount. Care should be exercised not to apply too large an amount of treated manure to soil, since applications heavier than 15 tons per acre are likely to injure some crops on certain soil types.

The use of properly baited fly traps as well as of kerosene-pyrethrum fly sprays is an important supplemental control measure. Instructions for making a thoroughly practical fly trap will be found in Farmers' Bulletin 734, Flytraps and Their Operation.,

Horseflies and Deerflies

The blood-sucking insects known as horseflies and deer flies are often very troublesome to horses. Their bites are painful, and when the insects are numerous, they draw considerable blood. They also act as carriers of anthrax, the Asiatic disease surra, and possibly other equine maladies.

There are many kinds of horseflies and deer flies of various sizes and colors (Fig. 1). Some are relatively small, not more than half an inch in length, while others are three times that size and very robust.

These pests are widely distributed in this country, being found in greatest number sin marshy or swampy areas and along streams, where they breed. The eggs are aid on plants growing in or over the water or on stones in streams. After hatching, the larvae drop into the water and burrow into the mud or gravel, where they feed on small, soft-bodied animals. After nearly a year they pupate in the moist soil near the water, and soon the adult insects emerge. The adults are strong, fast fliers and may be found several miles away from water, hut they are usually more abundant near it.

As the breeding habits suggest, control is very difficult. Draining swamps and seepage. areas along streams, deepening and straightening the edges of lakes and ponds, and preventing accumulations of waste irrigation water in low place in meadows tend to reduce the number of horseflies.

When these pests are abundant, animals in harness may be given some relief by the use of burlap coverings. Darkened sheds and smudges offer some protection to livestock not being worked. Horseflies are not easily repelled, and as the individual flies usually remain on the animals for only very short periods, fly sprays are of little value.

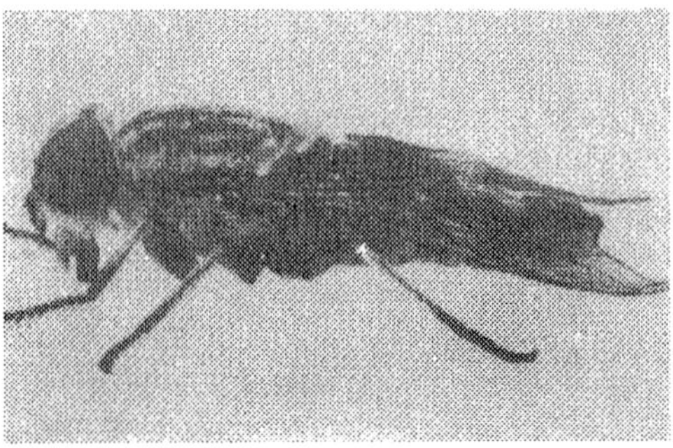

Fig. 1: A species of horsefly. Three times natural size.

Buffalo Gnats

Buffalo gnats, or blackflies, are pests of nearly all warm-blooded animals, but certain species prefer certain hosts. They are small, rather heavy-set, humpbacked flies, or gnats (Fig. 2). The bites they inflict on human beings are often very irritating; when there are many bites, the face and arms may become swollen; and severe generalized symptoms may result. Livestock are greatly annoyed by the bites of these insects. In severe outbreaks of the southern buffalo gnat in the lower Mississippi Valley many mules die, cattle, and horses are reduced in flesh, milk flow is cut, and the coats of the animals become rough and unsightly.

Buffalo gnats breed only in running water. The larvae attach themselves to sticks, logs, stones, and aquatic plants in the faster flowing parts of streams. Stones or dams over which water is rushing are often literally covered with the larvae, which, when full- grown, are from one-third to one-half inch in length. The larvae usually require several months to develop; then they pupate in cornucopia-like structures which they spin on rocks in the water. The gnats burst out of the pupa skins and in some way reach the surface of the rough water and fly off.

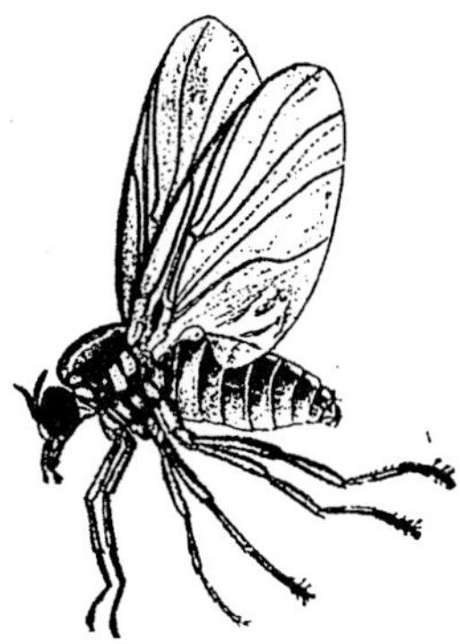

Fig. 2: Adult buffalo gnat, or blackfly. Much enlarged.

The adult females appear to require one or more meals of blood before eggs develop. These are laid in a gelatinous mass on stones or twigs at the water's surface or, as in the case of the southern buffalo gnat, are dropped singly on the water as the females dip to the surface from the swarm of gnats dancing over it. Bradley (2) has found that the eggs of the southern buffalo gnat sink to the bottom and do not hatch until the following spring when floods occur again. The eggs, of most species hatch in a few days.

The southern buffalo gnat usually appears in swarms in the lower Mississippi Valley during the first warm period of late winter or early spring. If the floods are widespread and the weather continues warm, tremendous numbers of gnats emerge. After a few weeks the gnats disappear, sometimes very suddenly.

The turkey gnat (*Eusimulium meridionale*), which usually appears later in the spring than does the southern buffalo gnat, attacks livestock to a limited extent but is especially destructive to poultry.

Preventing the breeding of the southern buffalo gnat is very difficult. Controlling floodwaters by holding them within dikes reduces the extent of breeding, and it is advisable to remove from streams logs, brush, and other obstructions to which the gnats can attach themselves. The removal of stones is sometimes practicable in more northerly streams where buffalo gnats breed. It is also helpful to install a series of dams to still the water where it normally ripples over stones.

In small streams near horse-breeding farms or vacation resorts where gnats are troublesome, emulsified pyrethrum concentrate may be used to kill the larvae. This material is very destructive to fish and other desirable aquatic life and therefore should be used only by an experienced person. If fish are present, nets must be placed across the stream to prevent then from drifting downstream with the treated water and thus being killed.

Smudges are commonly resorted to, especially in gnat areas in the South, and are helpful in protecting both livestock and human beings from severe attack.

Horses, mules, and cattle may be protected to some extent by being kept on high, open pastures as far from flooded streams as possible. Animals should be watched and removed to protected places promptly if a severe outbreak of gnats occurs, since the initial attack usually is the one that causes death.

Immunizing animals by inoculating them with "gnat extract," made from crushed and filtered gnats, has been tried by Georgevitch (3) with a species causing great losses in the Danube Valley. This method appears to have some promise, but further experimental work is necessary to determine its true value.

Many concoctions have been used as repellents to protect human beings and animals from gnats, but none is very satisfactory. One of those most commonly used on animals is crankcase oil with a little pine tar added. The difficulty most farmers experience with oils and greases is that after their continued use animals often some overheated when worked in the sun, the hair being shed in patches, and the skin sometimes being badly burned. In all effort to avoid these ill effects Bradley conducted some tests of non-oily materials and found the following formula to be promising as a protection against the southern buffalo gnat: Boil ½ pound of soap on 1 gallon of water and slowly add 6 ounces of pine-tar oil (specific gravity 1.065) while stirring vigorously; add 1 pint of this mixture to 2½ gallons of water; mop the animals with it in the morning and spray them lightly several times during the way. Another repellent, developed by Schwardt (9); is made by emulsifying 3 quarts of cylinder oil with 1 pint at fish-oil soap. This stock emulsion is diluted with 1 gallon of water and mopped or sprayed on the animals.

Fleas and Lice

Fleas, especially the human flea, sometimes worry, mules and horses considerably. These insects breed in barns, and their attacks frequently become so severe as to prevent horses and mules from standing in the barn even while eating.

Lice not infrequently become so numerous on horses and mules as make them unthrifity and rough-coated. Of the three kinds of lice found on equines, the bloodsucking species known as *Haematopinus asini* is the most injurious. This louse is about one-eighth of an inch in length and has an elongate head (Fig. 3). The other two species, known as *Trichodectes pilosus* and *T. parumpilosus,* have rounded heads and are usually yellowish or reddish brown. They have biting mouth parts and feed on skin scales. Sometimes they become incredibly numerous and seriously irritate horses, causing them to rub against objects, and to kick and stamp.

The species of lice mentioned confine their attacks to members of the horse family and remain on the host animal continuously. The young lice closely resemble the adults except that they are smaller and paler.

When removed from the host animal, the sucking lice are short-lived, living a maximum of 3 days under natural conditions. The biting lice, if kept on bunches of hair, may live for 10 days, but the majority of them die in 3 to 6 days. The eggs, or nits, are firmly attached to the horse's hair. The incubation period of the sucking louse is about 2 weeks and that of the biting lice is somewhat shorter. The sucking louse reaches maturity and the female begins laying eggs 11 or 12 days after hatching.

Lice are particularly abundant during the winter, when infestations may become very heavy before they are observed. Even when no control steps are taken, the lice diminish in numbers when

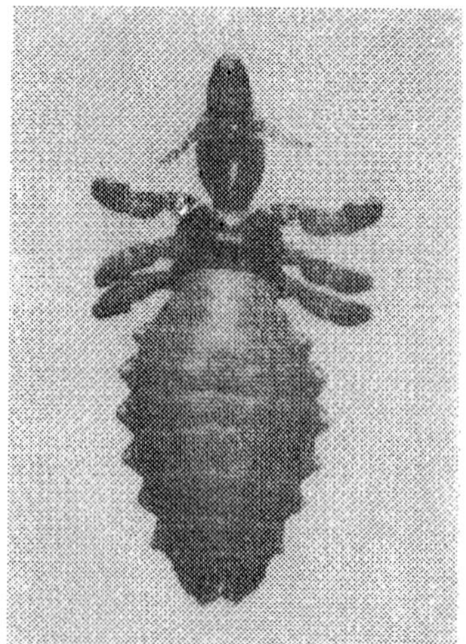

Fig. 3: Sucking louse of the horse and donkey. Much enlarged.

the hair is shed in the spring. However, a few of the parasites remain on the animals, usually in the mane and tail throughout the summer, and from these the infestation builds up again the next winter.

The presence of lice in large numbers is usually made known when the animal begins to rub itself against objects. The top of the tail is often made nearly bare in this way, and patches of hair are rubbed from the neck, shoulders, and flanks. Lice may pass from one animal to another by direct contact or by being rubbed off in corrals or barns.

A number of insecticides, if properly applied, are effective in killing lice, but since none of them will destroy the eggs, it is necessary to treat infested animals at least twice to delouse them entirely. The irregularity in the time required for eggs to hatch and for the lice to mature makes it difficult to set an exact period between dippings. Schwartz, Imes, and Wright state that "experience has shown that two dippings with an interval of 14 to 16 days usually can be depended on to control both sucking and biting lice.

Ticks

Several kinds of ticks attack horses and mules. One, called the tropical horse tick (*Dermacentor nitens*), prefers equines to other animals. The others attack various kinds of domestic and wild animals.

The tropical horse tick is found in the extreme southern part of Texas and in tropical America. It attaches itself mainly in the ears of the animal but may be found in the foretop and mane or elsewhere on the head and neck.

The Gulf coast tick, technically *Amblyomma maculatum*, in the adult stage attaches itself in the outer ear. The long beak of this tick makes a severe wound, and when a group of the ticks puncture an ear it becomes inflamed, thickened, and sore. Not infrequently screwworm flies are attracted to the infested ears, and their larvae burrow into the tissues. If the screwworms are killed in time the animal's life may be saved, but frequently cartilage is destroyed and the ears droop. When this occurs the animal is said to be gotch-eared.

The spinose ear tick (*Ornithodoros megnini*) attaches itself when in the seed-tick stage deep in the external ear. This tick is prevalent in the arid and semiarid Southwest. It is often present In such numbers as to fill the bottom of the ear and case much annoyance; Infested animals shake their heads, the ears and head are sensitive, and the animals are often hard to bridle. Heavy infestations, result in loss of flesh and an unthrifty appearance.

The seed ticks of this species molt and become nymphs in 7 to 12 days without leaving the ears. The nymphs become fully engorged (Fig. 4) and grow to about one-third of an inch long in 1 to 6 months; then they drop off the animal and crawl up a post, barn wall, or tree, where they find a hiding place and molt their spiny skins. The adults mate, and the females lay eggs in the hiding places, The eggs hatch in about 3 weeks, and the active seed ticks are then ready to attach themselves in the ears of an animal.

The two species of winter ticks, *Dermacentor albipictus* and *D. nigrolineatus* are widely distributed in this country. They appear to prefer horses and elk as hosts but also attack other domestic and wild animals. They frequently become so numerous, especially on range horses, as to cause extreme debility or even death. The seed ticks of these species become active late in the fall and attach themselves then or during warm periods in the winter or early spring. The ticks remain on the host during their two molts, and the females become engorged and drop off about 30 days after the seed ticks became attached.

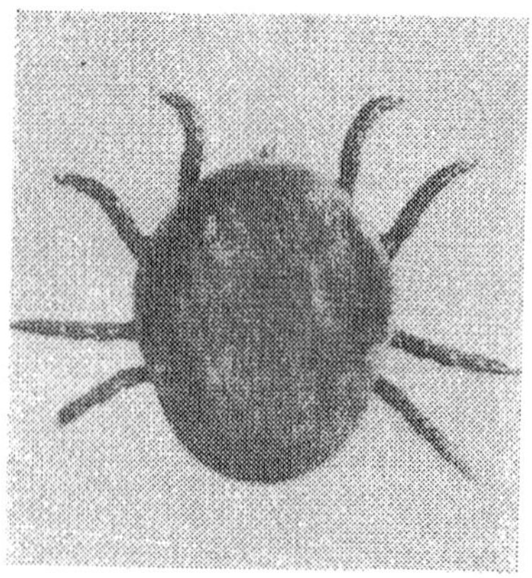

Fig. 4: Ear tick nymph, fully engorged. Much enlarged.

The cattle tick (*Boophilus annulatus*) often attacks horses and mules as well as bovines. Some individual animals appear to be very favorable hosts for this tick, while others are infested with few if any of them.

The American dog tick (*Dermacentor variabilis*) attaches itself to horses and human beings as well as to dogs and many other species of animals. On well-groomed horses this tick becomes attached mainly in the mane and tail and on the fetlocks. The ticks cause much irritation but are not known to carry any equine disease.

A number of other species of ticks are important as pests of horses in certain localities, among them the black-legged tick (*Ixodes ricinus scapularis*), the Pacific coast tick (*Dermacentor occidentalis*), the lone star tick (*Amblyomma americanum*), and the cayenne tick (*A. cajennense*).

Control measures for ticks must be fitted to the habits of the particular species. Horses infested with the ear tick and the Gulf coast tick may be freed of these pests by treating the ears with a mixture of 2 parts of pine tar and 1 part of cottonseed oil. In order to reach all the ear ticks, it is necessary to work the material into the ear or to break up the mass of ticks, as described by Imes (6). The liquid should not be allowed to run down the side of the face, as it may cause shedding of the hair. Applications every 2 to 4 weeks will usually keep either of these species under complete control. The same treatment is effective in controlling the tropical horse tick.

Dipping in an arsenical solution, is the most satisfactory way of destroying cattle ticks and other species that invest various parts of the animal other than the ears. The short period of engorgement and the genera host relations of such species as the cayenne tick, the lone star tick, and the black-legged tick make complete control by dipping impossible. The winter ticks are more resistant to arsenical dips than the cattle tick, and many of them survive dipping in the standard-strength arsenical solution. Two dippings at 14-day intervals in a solution containing 0.22 percent arsenic trioxide will destroy most of the ticks if the animal is not exposed to reinfestation. Mopping infested animals with a mixture of 2 ounces of finely ground derris containing 5 percent rotenone, 2 ounces of neutral soap, and 1 gallon of water would probably kill all the ticks with which the wash is brought in contact. This wash is also effective for the American dog tick. Clipping helps to keep ticks off saddle horses, and dusting derris or cube powder in the mane and fetlocks also helps to hold down infestations.

Literature Cited

(1) BISHOPP, F.C. (1939). DOMESTIC MOSQUITOES. U.S. Dept. Agr. Leaflet 186,8 pp., illus.

(2) BRADLEY, G.H. (1935). THE HATCHING OF EGGS OF THE SOUTHERN BUFFALO GNAT. Science 82: 277-278.

(3) GEORGEVITCH. JIVOIN (1923). NOUVELLES RECHERCHES SUR LA MOUCHE DE GOLOURATZ. [Prrris] Acad des Sci. Compt: Rend. 176: 1500-1502.

(4) HERMS, WILLIAM BRODBEOK, and GRAY, HAROLD FARNSWORTH (1940). MOSQUITO CONTROL. 317 pp., illus. New York.

(5) HOWARD, L.O., and BISHOPP, F.C. (1926). THE HOUSE FLY AND HOW TO SUPPRESS IT. U.S. Dept. Agr. Farmers' Bul. 1408,17 pp., illus., (Revised.)

(6) IMES, MARION (1918). THE SPINOSE EAR TICK. U.S. Dept. Agr. Farmers' Bul. 980, 8 pp., illus.

(7) KING, W.V., BRADLEY, G.H., and McNEEL, T.E. (1939). THE MOSQUITOES OF THE SOUTHEASTERN STATES. U.S. Dept. Agr. Misc. Pub. 336, 91 pp., illus.

(8) RANSOM, B.H. (1913). THE LIFE HISTORY OF HABRONEMA MUSCAE (CARIER), A PARASITE OF THE HORSE TRANSMI1TED BY THE HOUSE FLY. U.S. Bur. Anim. Indus. 163, 36 pp., illus.

(9) SOHWARDT, H.H. (1935). LUBRICATING OIL EMULSION AS A BUFFALO GNAT REPELLENT. Kans. Ent. Soc. Jour. 8: 141.

(10) SCHWARTZ, BENJAMIN, IMES, MARION, and WRIGHT, W.W. (1936). PARASITES AND PARISITIC DISEASES OF HORSES. U.S. Dept. Agr. Cir. 148, 55 pp., illus. (Revised).

INDEX